UNINTENTIONAL
SUICIDE

UNINTENTIONAL SUICIDE

A Doctor's Guide to Preventing Disease

Tim Loy, MD

LANGDON STREET PRESS • MINNEAPOLIS

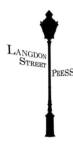

Langdon Street Press
322 First Avenue N, 5th floor
Minneapolis, MN 55401
612.455.2293
www.langdonstreetpress.com

ISBN-13: 978-1-63413-746-1
LCCN: 2015913203

Distributed by Itasca Books

Book Design by MK Ross

Printed in the United States of America

CONTENTS

ACKNOWLEDGMENTS

This project would never have been completed if I had not received help from many people. I thank Michele Smith and Carolyn Lane for their excellent clerical help and for typing the first draft of the manuscript. I thank Tim Perkins for his help in finding autopsy photographs for illustrations. Nick Libla, Sarah Robertson, and Van Nguyen saved me many times when I ran into computer difficulties. I am indebted to the many people who donated photographs or allowed me to reprint them in this book. They are acknowledged in the figure legends. Other images were provided by the author. Sharon Stack graciously helped me produce figures 1-12 and 1-13. Tyson Loy, one of my handsome sons, modeled for the figures in the exercise chapter. Mitzi Loy, my wonderful wife, proofread the manuscript and offered many helpful suggestions. Finally, I thank Kate Ankofski of Langdon Street Press for her outstanding editing and insights.

INTRODUCTION

A great tragedy is occurring. Millions of people are dying prematurely. These people are killing themselves and they don't even know it.

For twenty-four years, I worked as a surgical pathologist at the University of Missouri. I read biopsies for a living. Each day, I diagnosed terrible diseases. Each day I was reminded that many of these were self-inflicted. Though the causes of these diseases are well-known, they are often ignored, time and time again.

As I gathered the information included in this book, it became clear that widely adopted lifestyle changes would do more to improve health and save lives than any recent "wonder drug." The challenge was how to help others see the tremendous health benefits they could reap through simple lifestyle changes. I saw two opportunities for meeting this challenge: encourage the medical profession to put more emphasis on disease prevention, and directly reach out to the general public.

I recently accepted an offer to join the faculty of Ross University, one of the world's largest medical schools. I hope that this position will enable me to teach more doctors to encourage their patients to adopt better health habits. In the meantime, this book is my effort to reach out to the general public, and echoes the voice inside me that wants to scream, *Quit killing yourselves!*

The relationship between lifestyle and disease has been well established. A twenty-four-year Harvard study of over 77,000 women found that 55 percent of their deaths could be attributed to smoking, obesity, a lack of physical activity, or a low-quality diet (1). Similarly, a Cambridge study has suggested that a healthy lifestyle could add fourteen years to our lives (2).

The top five causes of death in the United States are heart disease, cancer, stroke, chronic lung disease, and accidents (3). Fortunately, most of these deaths could be prevented.

Atherosclerosis, a disease of the arteries, causes the vast majority of heart disease and strokes. In the Western world, atherosclerosis often starts in childhood and is almost always present in adults. Eventually, atherosclerosis closes the affected artery, causing diseases such as heart attacks, strokes, and gangrene, and accounts for about one-third of the deaths in our society. The good news is that 90 percent of the diseases caused by atherosclerosis could be prevented through lifestyle changes.

Cancer currently develops in about half of men and a third of women in the United States. It causes nearly one-quarter of the deaths in our population. And yet over two-thirds of cancer could be avoided through lifestyle changes.

Chronic lung disease is the third-most-common killer in our country, causing about 5 percent of deaths. Ninety percent of chronic lung disease could be prevented if people quit smoking.

Accidents also cause about 5 percent of US deaths; here, too, most could be avoided through lifestyle changes.

Surgical pathologists have a rare opportunity to see and study the diseases in our society. While this job is fascinating, it can also be depressing. At times I have thought that if the general population could see what I see, they might be more likely to make changes in their day-to-day lives. It is very common for patients to make lifestyle changes *after* they develop symptoms of a serious disease. For example, I have commonly seen biopsies of lung cancer from patients who stopped smoking the previous week. Symptoms such as coughing up blood get their attention and make them realize that their smoking really could cause them to develop cancer. Unfortunately, such lifestyle changes often occur too late to save them. I hope that by giving you a personal tour of these diseases, I can help you and your loved ones make choices that can prevent disease *before* it is too late.

Unintentional Suicide is your glimpse into the destruction caused by the most prevalent diseases in our society—destruction that is likely to affect you or your loved ones in the future, if it hasn't already affected you in the past. The purpose of sharing my experience with you is to guide you toward a lifestyle that is easy to maintain, and to keep you as healthy as possible, for as long as possible.

The first portion of the book delves into everything you need to know about the illnesses causing so many of the deaths in our society—the top five killers, as well as other diseases becoming more prevalent each year. Many illustrations, including graphic photographs, are included in these chapters. While some may find these images offensive, my intention is only to depict the brutal devastation caused by these maladies. The remainder of the book examines lifestyle choices with practical suggestions to improve your health—starting now.

By choosing to read this book, you are making an important step toward wellness. I wish you well on your journey.

—Tim Loy, MD, March 2014

References:

1. van Dam et al. "Combined Impact of Lifestyle Factors on Mortality: Prospective Cohort Study in US Women." *British Medical Journal* 337 (2008): a1440.

2. Kwah et al. "Combined Impact of Health Behaviours and Mortality in Men and Women: The EPIC-Norfolk Prospective Population Study." PLOS Medicine 5, no. 1 (2008): e12.

3. Centers for Disease Control and Prevention. "FastStats Deaths and Mortality." Atlanta, GA: CDC, June 2010. www.cdc.gov/nchs/fastats/deaths.htm.

4. Thrasher, JF et al. "Cigarette Warning Label Policy Alternatives and Smoking-Related Health Disparities. American Journal of Preventive Medicine, Volume 43, Issue 6 , 590–600

PART I

THE COMMON KILLERS

1: ATHEROSCLEROSIS

Atherosclerosis is the leading cause of death in the Western world. In the United States alone, atherosclerosis kills about 800,000 people per year—over 2,000 Americans per day—with an annual cost to the American people of about $234 billion (1). Most of these deaths could be prevented.

BACKGROUND INFORMATION

Each day our heart beats 100,000 times to pump blood through 100,000 miles of vessels in order to supply 100 trillion cells with oxygen and nutrients. In short, our circulatory system is amazing. Most of our vessels are thin-walled capillaries through which the exchange of nutrients, oxygen, and waste products occur. Arteries carry blood from the heart to the capillary bed, while veins return the blood from the capillary bed to the heart.

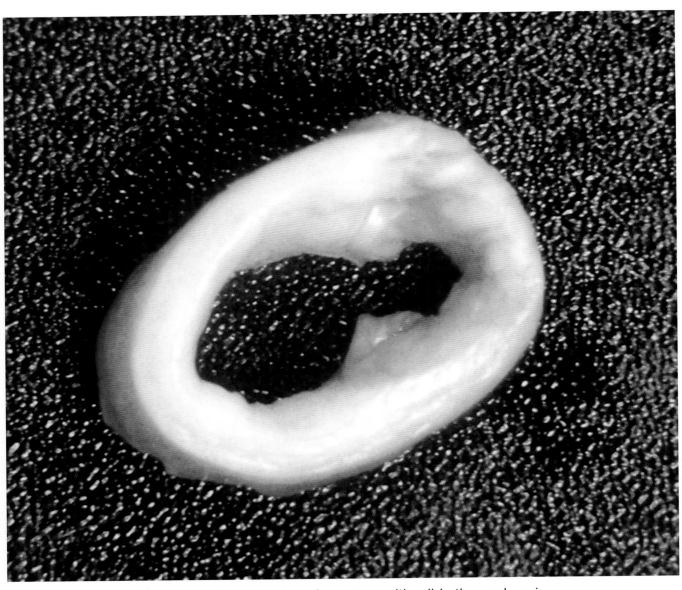

Figure 1-1: Cross section of an artery with mild atherosclerosis.
Photo courtesy of Scotty Holly, MD.

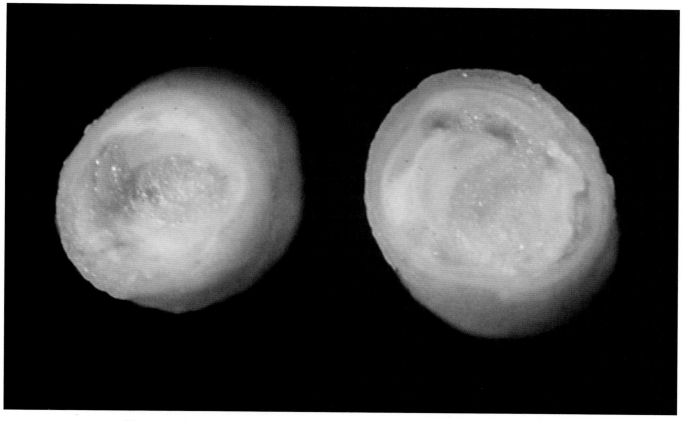

Figure 1-2: Cross sections of an artery clogged by atherosclerosis.
Photo courtesy of Douglas Miller, MD.

Atherosclerosis affects arteries, eventually clogging them up (Figs. 1-1, 1-2). As a result, blood can no longer get through the clogged arteries; whichever body part is supplied by that artery dies. "Infarct" is a medical term used to describe this death of a body part due to the lack of blood supply. If the clogged artery was a coronary artery supplying the heart muscle (myocardium), the person suffers a myocardial infarction, commonly known as a heart attack (Figs. 1-3 to 1-5).

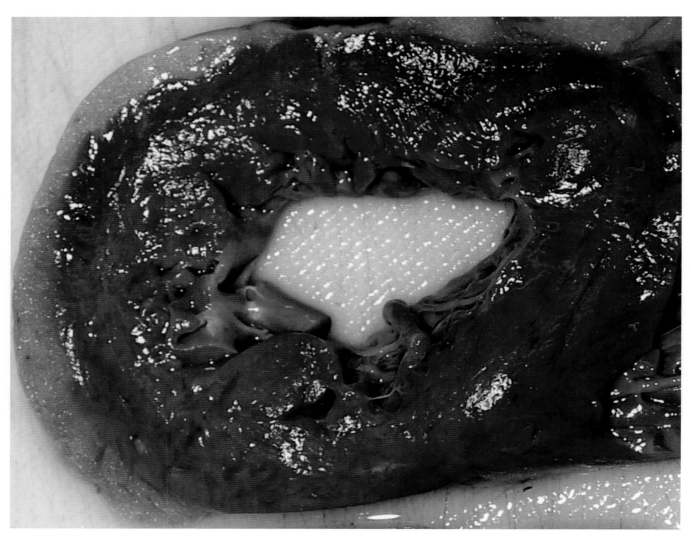

Figure 1-3: Cross section of normal left ventricle of heart.

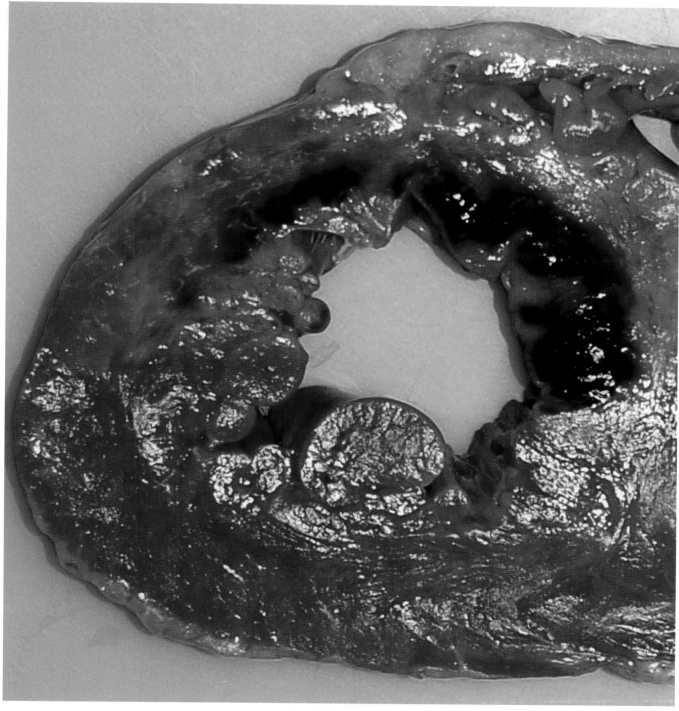

Figure 1-4: Recent myocardial infarction (red hemorrhagic area).

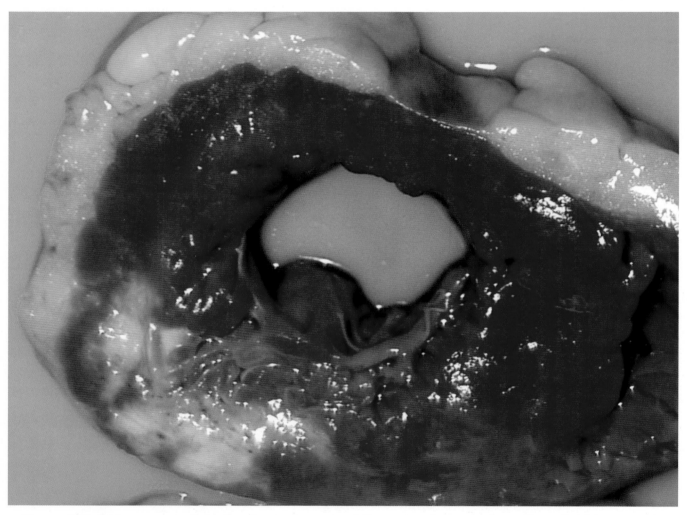

Figure 1-5: Older myocardial infarction, where dead tissue has been replaced by a light tan scar, is seen next to a mottled red-tan more recent infarction (bottom center).

If the clogged artery was supplying a portion of the brain, the person suffers a cerebral infarction, otherwise known as a stroke (Figs. 1-6 to 1-8).

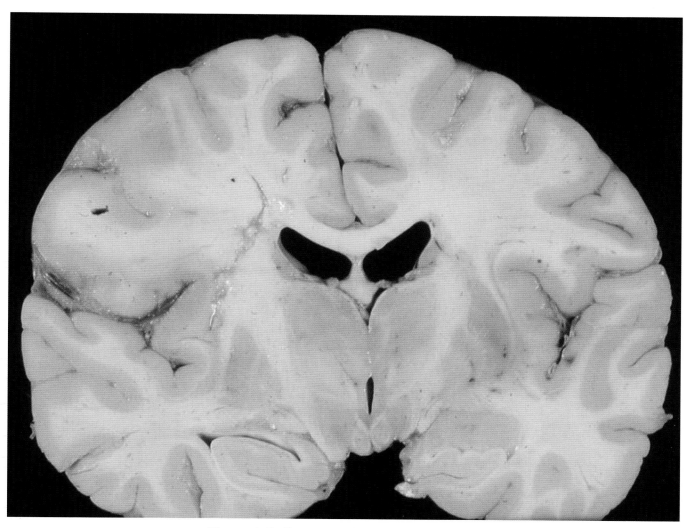

Figure 1-6: Cross section of normal brain.
Photo courtesy of Douglas Miller, MD.

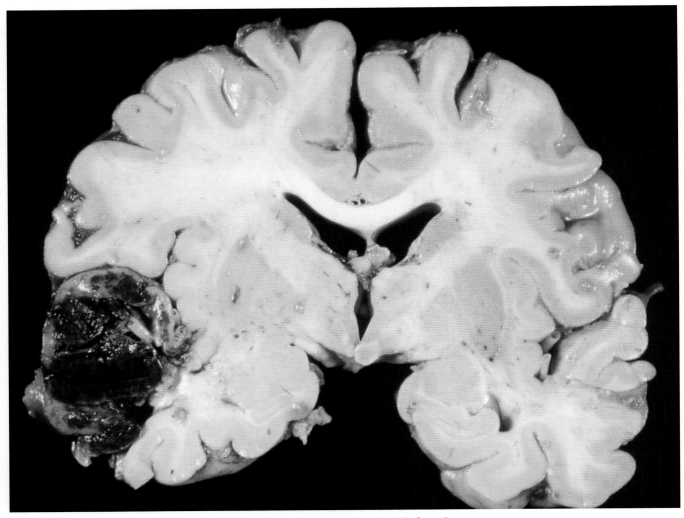

Figure 1-7: Recent cerebral infarction.
Photo courtesy of Douglas Miller, MD.

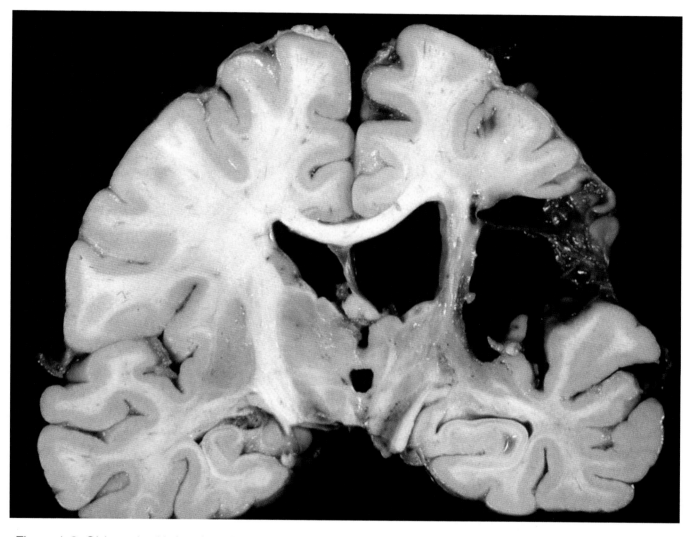

Figure 1-8: Old cerebral infarction. The dead tissue has been removed by the body, leaving an empty space. Photo courtesy of Douglas Miller, MD.

The clogging of arteries that supply blood to a limb leads to death (necrosis) of that limb—in other words, gangrene (Fig. 1-9).

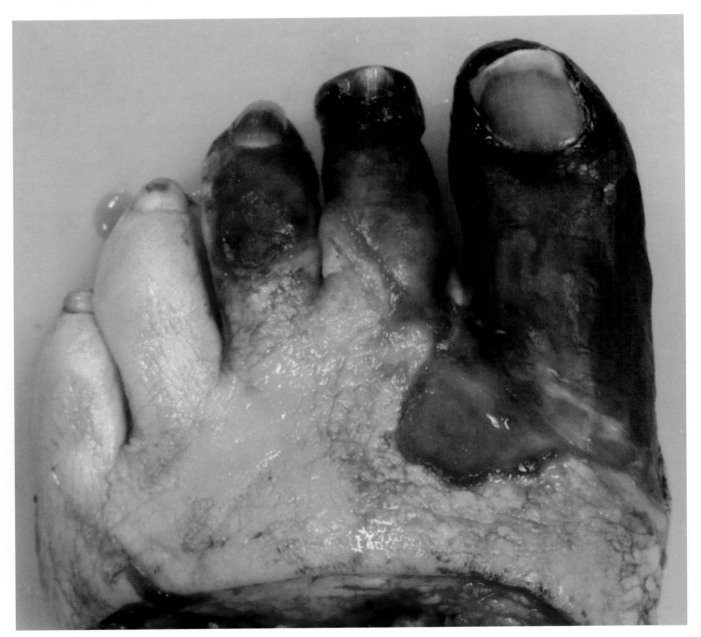

Figure 1-9: Gangrene.

Figure 1-10 shows what a normal artery looks like under the microscope.

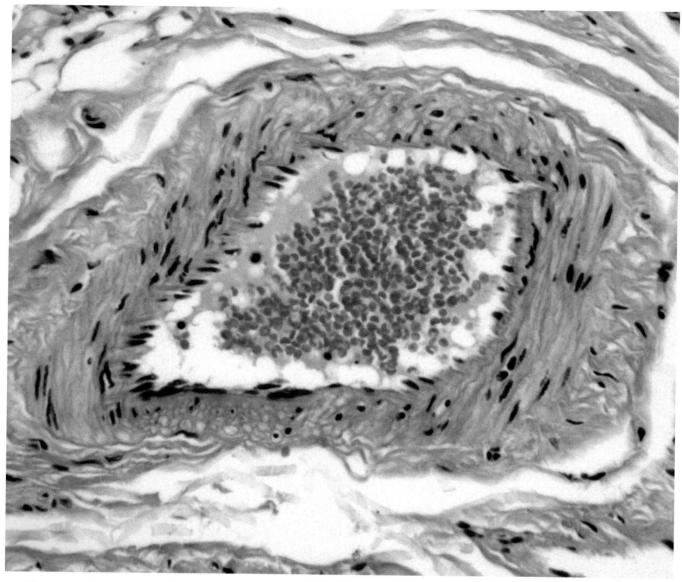

Figure 1-10: Normal artery. Note red blood cells in the lumen and inner lining of endothelial cells.

Note the single layer of thin cells lining the lumen. These cells are called endothelial cells and are very important in the development of atherosclerosis.

While atherosclerosis is not completely understood, it is thought that it starts with chronic injury to endothelial cells (2). This cellular injury may be due to high blood pressure, chemicals from cigarette smoke, or other toxic substances in the blood. The injured endothelial cells become leaky, allowing fatty substances in the blood called low-density lipoproteins (LDLs) to accumulate in the wall of the artery. Accumulation of these lipids in the wall causes the lumen to narrow, which leads to decreased blood flow through the artery. Inflammation caused by the injured endothelial cells and lipid accumulation causes scarring, which further narrows the lumen of the artery. Early atherosclerotic lesions are, however, reversible, as cholesterol deposited by the LDLs can be removed by high-density lipoproteins (HDLs) and returned to the bloodstream for disposal. However, once significant scarring and muscle proliferation have occurred, the artery will have been permanently narrowed (Fig. 1-11). Advanced cases of atherosclerosis may show calcification and even bone formation.

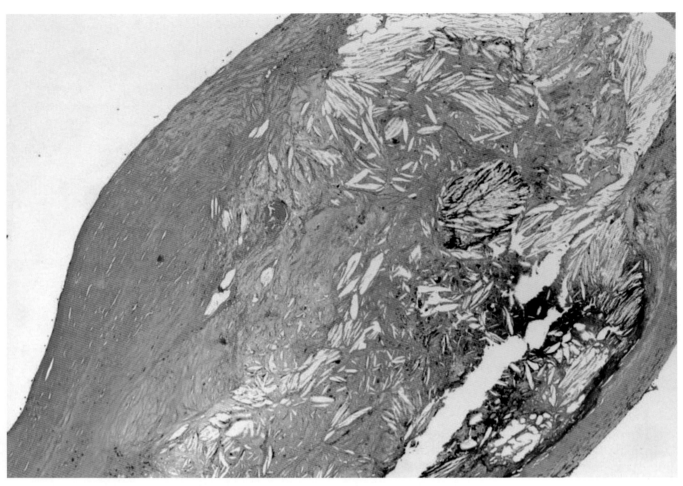

Figure 1-11: Atherosclerotic plaque.
The needle-shaped clear spaces represent cholesterol/lipid deposits.

Some of the risk factors for atherosclerosis, including family history, genetic abnormalities, male gender, or increasing age obviously cannot be modified. But hyperlipidemia, hypertension, cigarette smoking, and diabetes are all major factors that you have the power to control (2). Recent evidence suggests that high blood levels of homocysteine, a substance formed when protein is broken down, may be another important risk factor. A recent study found that 92.5 percent of US adults had at least one preventable risk factor for atherosclerosis (1).

HYPERLIPIDEMIA

Hyperlipidemia refers to high levels of cholesterol and/or triglycerides in the blood. Hypercholesterolemia (high blood cholesterol levels) is a major risk factor for atherosclerosis. Elevated cholesterol can stimulate atherosclerosis even if other risk factors are absent. Patients affected with familial hypercholesterolemia, a condition associated with blood cholesterol levels of over 1000 mg/dl, develop atherosclerosis at an early age, and often experience heart attacks during their teenage years. Conversely, atherosclerosis is very rare in patients with blood cholesterol levels less than 150 mg/dl (3). Fortunately, most people can significantly lower their cholesterol levels through simple lifestyle changes.

To understand hypercholesterolemia, let's first review normal cholesterol metabolism. Cholesterol is used by our bodies to make numerous essential substances such as hormones, cell membranes, and bile. Cholesterol is not water soluble and must be carried in the blood by lipoproteins. Most of the circulating cholesterol is attached to low-density lipoproteins (LDLs). To our arteries, LDL cholesterol is the bad type of cholesterol that is deposited into arteries, increasing atherosclerosis. High-density lipoprotein (HDL) is the good type, as it removes cholesterol from the arteries and helps to reverse atherosclerosis.

The major sources of cholesterol in our blood are dietary cholesterol—cholesterol that we eat—and endogenous cholesterol, which is produced by our liver. Dietary cholesterol only comes from animal sources and can be essentially eliminated by a vegetarian diet. The liver plays a central role in regulating the body's cholesterol balance. It removes cholesterol from the blood and makes new cholesterol as needed. Fat in our diet can affect how the liver handles cholesterol and cholesterol levels in the blood. While the diet's effect on the liver is complicated, here are some simplistic general rules: Unsaturated fat in the diet tends to lower blood LDLs by increasing cholesterol uptake by the liver. Saturated fat in the diet will raise blood LDLs by decreasing cholesterol uptake by the liver. Trans fats increase blood LDLs by causing the liver to make more cholesterol. To make matters worse, trans fats also lower HDLs. Endogenous cholesterol produced by the liver is used to make very low-density lipoproteins (VLDL), which are used to transport triglycerides and are later converted to LDLs (4). Since LDLs are the main source of the cholesterol deposited in atherosclerosis, much attention has been given to how our diet affects LDL levels. Increased consumption of cholesterol, saturated fat, and trans fats have all been considered risk factors for high blood LDL levels. These dietary factors tend to work together, and increased consumption of cholesterol alone may not elevate LDLs if the intake of saturated fat and trans fat is low. This has led to the controversial viewpoint of some that dietary cholesterol is no longer a substance of concern.

The liver also makes bile from cholesterol that is used to emulsify dietary fat. Bile is released from the gallbladder into the intestine after a fatty meal. It is later reabsorbed by the intestine. Normally our bile circulates in this cycle five to ten times per day; approximately 95 percent of the bile is reabsorbed in each cycle. This bile cycle is important, as it represents an excellent opportunity to get rid of excess cholesterol.

Dietary soluble fiber in the intestine binds bile and prevents intestinal reabsorption. Good dietary sources of soluble fiber include beans, lentils, peas, oats, and fruit. Dietary supplements rich in soluble fiber include psyllium, which you can find in your grocery store as Metamucil, and wheat dextrin, which is found in Benefiber. The bile with its cholesterol bound to fiber is later excreted with the feces (5). Fecal excretion of bile-associated cholesterol is the only effective way to remove excess cholesterol from the body (6).

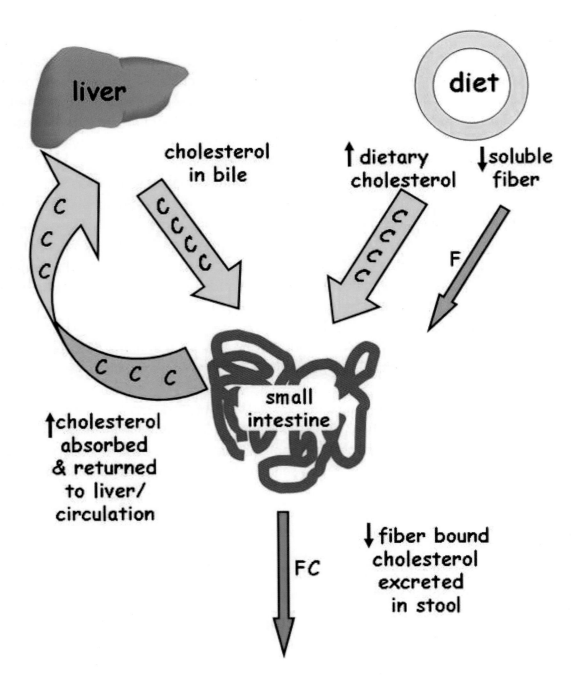

Figure 1-12. Cholesterol cycle with typical western diet.
Figure courtesy of Sharon Stack, PhD.

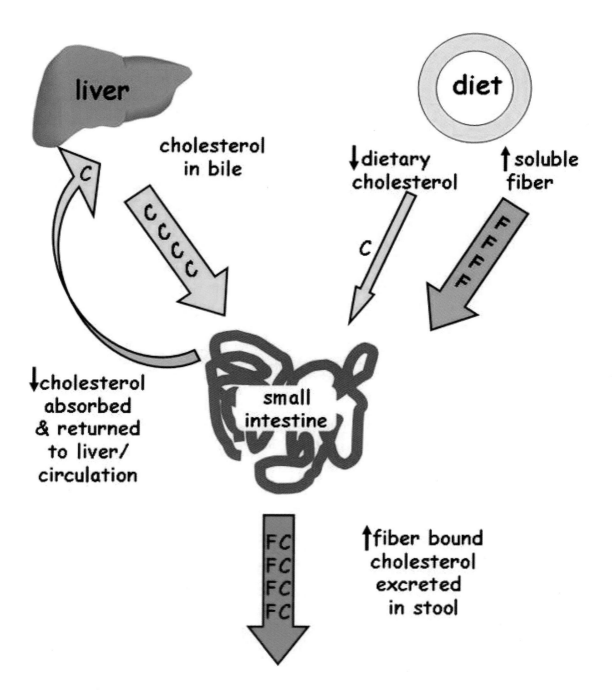

Figure 1-13. Cholesterol cycle with high fiber plant based diet.
Figure courtesy of Sharon Stack, PhD.

A typical Western diet with high dietary saturated fat, high dietary cholesterol, and low dietary soluble fiber encourages hypercholesterolemia (Fig. 1-12), whereas a plant-based diet with low cholesterol and high soluble fiber leads to lower cholesterol levels (Fig. 1-13). Serum cholesterol can also be lowered by drugs that decrease the liver's production of cholesterol. However, these drugs can have significant side effects such as muscle and liver damage. They should only be taken after lifestyle changes fail to achieve desirable cholesterol levels.

Lowering high cholesterol is a powerful way to decrease the risk of a heart attack. Studies have found that even a 10 percent reduction in total serum cholesterol levels decreases the risk of a heart attack up to 38 percent (7). Lifestyle changes specifically targeting levels of LDLs and HDLs are even more beneficial. Basically, you want your LDLs to be as low as possible and your HDLs to be as high as possible. Many experts believe that atherosclerosis could be virtually eliminated if people kept their LDL cholesterol below 70 mg/dl (8). This can be achieved with simple lifestyle changes including a plant-based diet rich in soluble fiber. Notably, some doctors think that low levels of HDLs may contribute to atherosclerosis even more than high levels of LDLs (9).

Aerobic exercise is a good way to increase high-density lipoproteins. It appears that HDL elevation is more dependent on the duration of the exercise sessions than on their intensity or frequency. HDLs begin to rise once you've exercised aerobically for 120 minutes per week. Once exercise sessions reach thirty minutes, each additional ten minutes of exercise is associated with a 1.4 mg/dl increase in HDL (10). While moderate alcohol consumption—defined as one drink containing one-half ounce of ethanol per day—may also increase HDLs, the risks associated with alcohol may outweigh its benefits. (See chapter 8 for an in-depth look at alcohol's pros and cons.)

TRIGLYCERIDES

Hypertriglyceridemia, or high levels of blood triglycerides, is an independent risk factor for atherosclerosis (12). Triglycerides are the chief form of fat in the diet as well as the body's preferred method of storing fat. High triglyceride levels in the blood are associated with obesity, excess calorie consumption, and alcohol consumption. High-fat foods, particularly saturated fats and simple sugars, can raise blood triglycerides. Weight reduction, exercise, and omega-3 fatty acids found primarily in fish can lower triglyceride levels.

HYPERTENSION (HIGH BLOOD PRESSURE)

High blood pressure is a major risk factor of atherosclerosis, no matter your age. Hypertension is responsible for more than a five-fold increased risk of coronary artery disease (2). High blood pressure causes atherosclerosis by injuring the endothelial cells lining the arteries. Risk factors for hypertension include stress, obesity, smoking, physical inactivity, and a high-sodium, low-potassium diet. Nearly 30 percent of US adults suffer from high blood pressure, primarily as a result of obesity. Even minor reductions in blood pressure can reap great benefits: it has been estimated that a 9.5 percent decrease in sodium consumption by US adults aged forty to eight-five years would prevent 513,885 strokes and 480,358 heart attacks over their lifetime and save more than $32 billion in medical costs (13).

CIGARETTE SMOKING

Smoking is another well-established risk factor for atherosclerosis. Smokers have up to a 200 percent increased death rate from heart attacks (2). The increased risk of atherosclerosis in smokers is likely due to damaged endothelial cells from smoking-related toxins.

DIABETES

The high blood sugar levels associated with diabetes are toxic to endothelial cells. Diabetes is also associated with high blood cholesterol levels. These factors lead to a markedly increased predisposition to atherosclerosis. Diabetics experience twice as many heart attacks as nondiabetics, and have a hundredfold increased chance of developing gangrene in the legs, feet, or toes. (2). Most, but not all, cases of diabetes are caused by obesity.

HOMOCYSTEINE

Homocysteine is an amino acid that is normally produced in our bodies through the metabolism of proteins in our diet. Our bodies normally break down homocysteine with metabolic pathways using folate, vitamin B12, vitamin B6, and betaine. Deficiencies in these vitamins can lead to elevated blood levels of homocysteine.

Elevated homocysteine contributes to atherosclerosis through direct damage to endothelial cells. Elevated homcysteine may also encourage arterial blockage by promoting clots. Patients with homocystinuria, a rare condition associated with very high homocysteine levels (over one hundred micromoles per liter) often develop severe atherosclerosis as teenagers. Homocystinuria is transmitted by a recessive gene; as a result, a child is only susceptible to the disease if both parents carry the gene. About 1 percent of the population carries a single gene for homocystinuria; these individuals have milder elevations of homocysteine than patients with both genes for the disease. Lowering homocysteine levels has been proven to lower the risk of atherosclerosis in people with homocystinuria. It is still unknown whether people with mildly elevated homocysteine (about 10 to 12 micromoles per liter) also benefit from lowering their homocysteine levels.

As we've already discussed, studies have shown that diets rich in folate, vitamin B6, vitamin B12, and betaine can lower homocysteine levels. Good dietary sources of folate and vitamin B6 include fruits, vegetables, beans, and cereals. Vitamin B12 is found in meat, fish, and dairy products. Gastric atrophy, a common problem as we age, refers to the thinning of the stomach lining, which can lead to poor absorption of vitamin B12 as well as elevated homocysteine levels. Vitamin B12 supplements have been recommended for people over age fifty and for vegetarians of any age. Major food sources of betaine include wheat germ, whole wheat, wheat bran, spinach, and beets.

PERSONAL OBSERVATIONS

I have a strong family history of atherosclerosis and heart disease. My grandfather developed heart disease in his forties and had a fatal heart attack ten years later. My father suffered but survived a large heart attack when he was fifty-two.

Throughout my adult life, I have always been considered a health nut. I've tried to eat healthy, exercise avidly, and abstain from alcohol, and I have never smoked. After my doctor suggested that I have my cholesterol checked at age forty-nine, I was surprised to find that it was 195 mg/dl with an HDL of 57 and an LDL of 126. Though these are considered desirable numbers, they are still at a level that supports the development of atherosclerosis.

I switched to a low-fat, vegetarian diet and used soluble fiber supplements. Three months later, my labs came back: cholesterol 152 mg/dl, HDL 49 mg/dl, and LDL 95 mg/dl. Good numbers, but still not good enough. When I learned that too little fat in my diet could lower HDLs—the opposite effect of what I wanted—I added fish to my diet and increased my aerobic exercise.

Two years after my initial cholesterol readings, my numbers revealed my efforts had paid off: cholesterol 140mg/dl, HDL 67 mg/dl, and LDL 67 mg/dl. These lipid levels are associated with a very low risk of atherosclerosis.

Recently, Laurence Sperling, MD, who is the director of Heart Disease Prevention at Emory University and president of the American Society of Preventive Cardiology, visited Ross University. He gave a presentation that showed that 90 percent of cardiovascular disease could be prevented through lifestyle changes. My story supports his data. Through simple lifestyle changes, you too can significantly reduce your risk of suffering from this killer disease.

RECOMMENDATIONS FOR DECREASING YOUR RISK OF ATHEROSCLEROSIS

1. Eat a plant-based diet high in soluble fiber and low in cholesterol and saturated fat.
2. Shoot for ten servings a day of fruits and vegetables.
3. Eat omega-3–rich fish such as salmon twice a week.
4. Avoid excess salt and sugar by reducing intake of processed junk foods.
5. Quit smoking.
6. Exercise.
7. Lose as much weight as is necessary to reach your ideal body weight.
8. If you're a vegetarian, take a vitamin B12 supplement daily.
9. If applicable, seek medical treatment for hypertension and diabetes—the sooner, the better.

If these recommendations were followed, millions of deaths from atherosclerosis could be prevented.

REFERENCES:

1. Ford et al. "Trends in the Prevalence of Low Risk Factor Burden for Cardiovascular Disease among United States Adults." *Circulation* 120 (2009): 1181–88.

2. Schoen FJ. "Blood Vessels." In *Robbins and Cotran Pathologic Basis of Disease*, 7th ed., edited by Kumar et al, 511–32. Philadelphia, PA: Elsevier Saunders, 2005.

3. Roberts WC. "Preventing and Arresting Coronary Atherosclerosis." *American Heart Journal* 130, no. 3 pt 1 (September 1995): 580–600.

4. Ginsberg HN, Goldberg IJ. "Disorders of Lipoprotein Metabolism." In *Harrison's Principles of Internal Medicine*, 14th ed., edited by Fauci et al, 2141. St. Louis, MO: McGraw-Hill, 1998.

5. Rolfes SR, Pinna K, Whitney E. *Understanding Normal and Clinical Nutrition.* 7th ed. Belmont, CA: Thomson Wadsworth, 2006: 150.

6. Crawford JM. "Liver and Biliary Tract." In *Robbins and Cotran Pathologic Basis of Disease*, 7th ed., edited by Kumar et al, 887. Philadelphia, PA: Elsevier Saunders, 2005.

7. Law MR, Wald NJ, Thompson SG. "By How Much and How Quickly Does Reduction in Serum Cholesterol Concentration Lower Risk of Ischaemic Heart Disease?" *British Medical Journal* 308 (1994): 367–72.

8. Roberts WC. "The Cause of Atherosclerosis." *Nutrition in Clinical Practice* 23 (2008): 464–67.

9. Cardenas et al. "The Importance of Recognizing and Treating Low Levels of High-Density Lipoprotein Cholesterol: A New Era in Atherosclerosis Management." *Reviews in Cardiovascular Medicine* 9, no. 4 (2008): 239–58.

10. Kodama et al. "Effect of Aerobic Exercise Training on Serum Levels of High- Density Lipoprotein Cholesterol." *Archives of Internal Medicine* 167 (2007): 999–1008.

11. Digby JE, Lee JMS, Choudhury RP. "Nicotinic Acid and the Prevention of Coronary Artery Disease." *Current Opinion in Lipidology* 20, no. 4 (2009): 321–26.

12. Hennig et al. "High-Energy Diets, Fatty Acids and Endothelial Cell Function: Implications for Atherosclerosis." *Journal of the American College of Nutrition* 20, no. 2 (2001): 97–105.

13. Smith-Spangler et al. "Population Strategies to Decrease Sodium Intake and the Burden of Cardiovascular Disease: A Cost-Effectiveness Analysis." *Annals of Internal Medicine* (March 2010).

2.0: CANCER

Cancer is the most feared disease in our society, and it may soon surpass atherosclerosis as the world's top killer. Worldwide, about 12 million new cancer cases are diagnosed and about 7.6 million people die of the disease each year. It is estimated that nearly 1.6 million new cancer cases were diagnosed in the United States in 2011. Currently, half of the men and one-third of the women in the US develop cancer over the course of their lifetime (1). A majority of these cancers could have been prevented.

BACKGROUND INFORMATION

Our cells have an amazingly elaborate set of controls to regulate cell proliferation. Consider the events that occur when you sustain a minor injury, such as cutting your finger. Tissue damage leads to the release of a variety of substances that stimulate the growth of many types of cells. Without you even having to think about it, fibroblasts make collagen, vessels rapidly proliferate, and epithelial cells multiply to repair the skin damaged by the injury. After healing has occurred, these cell types cease to proliferate.

Cells make proteins, which allow all these wonderful things to happen. The blueprint for these proteins is contained in DNA stored in the nucleus of each cell. DNA sequences—otherwise known as genes—encode proteins, which regulate all bodily functions, including cell proliferation. Each time a cell divides, the entire DNA sequence is replicated. Some of the genes in the DNA code lead to the formation of substances that ensure that the encoded information remains intact. Other genes encode for proteins that are responsible for repairing damaged DNA. Another type regulates programmed cell death, or apoptosis, which causes old or damaged cells to expire.

This may seem like an unnecessary science lesson, but as you'll see, this information is needed when trying to understand how cancers develop.

PATHOLOGY

About 10 billion of our cells die and are replaced each day. That means our DNA is replicated 10 billion times each day. DNA replication is amazingly accurate; however, mistakes can occur. Environmental factors such as radiation from the sun, chemicals in our food, and toxins in cigarette smoke damage the DNA of about 1 million cells per day. Factors that cause DNA damage or stimulate the growth of tumor cells are called carcinogens. Replication errors and carcinogens can lead to changes in the DNA coding for genes regulating cell functions. These changes in the DNA are called mutations.

Tumors occur when a mutation in the DNA leads to a proliferation of cells with altered genes regulating cell proliferation. Cancer cells have their proliferation genes permanently switched on. Many cancers also have gene mutations that prevent natural cell death from occurring. The result is an uncontrolled proliferation of cells that can spread throughout the body, eventually causing death.

The body has a complex system of defense mechanisms that fight against cancer formation. DNA mutations are usually repaired. Even if the DNA is not repaired, most mutated cells are killed by the immune system or natural cell death. With chronic exposure to carcinogens, large numbers of mutated cells can develop, which can overwhelm the body's defenses and result in cancer. If you limit your exposure to carcinogens, you can significantly reduce your cancer risk. Tips for avoiding carcinogens causing specific types of cancer will be given in the remainder of this chapter.

Tumors can form in every organ and from every type of cell found in the body; hundreds of different tumor types exist. Malignant tumors occur when mutations lead to a proliferation of cells that can invade adjacent normal tissues and spread, or metastasize, to other parts of the body through the bloodstream or lymphatic system (Figs. 2.0-1 to 2.0-3).

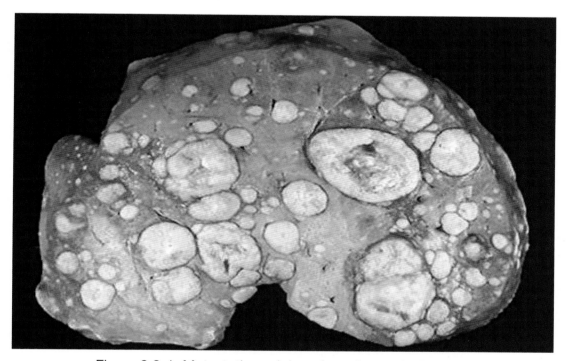

Figure 2.0-1: Metastatic nodules of carcinoma in the liver.
Photo courtesy of Alberto Diaz-Arias, MD.

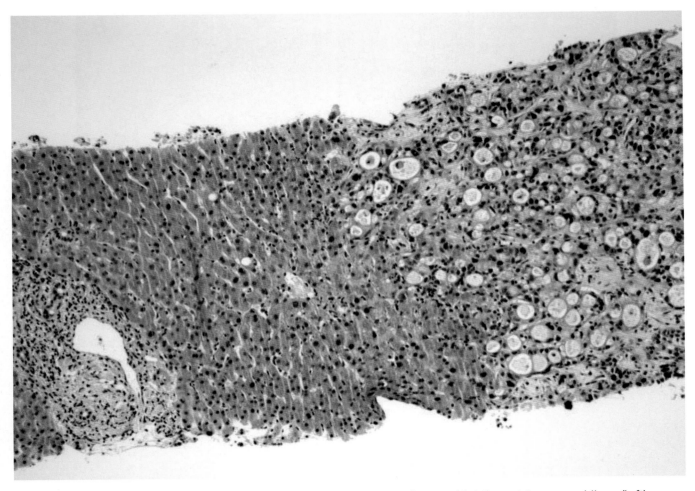

Figure 2.0-2: Liver biopsy showing metastatic adenocarcinoma (right) next to normal liver (left).

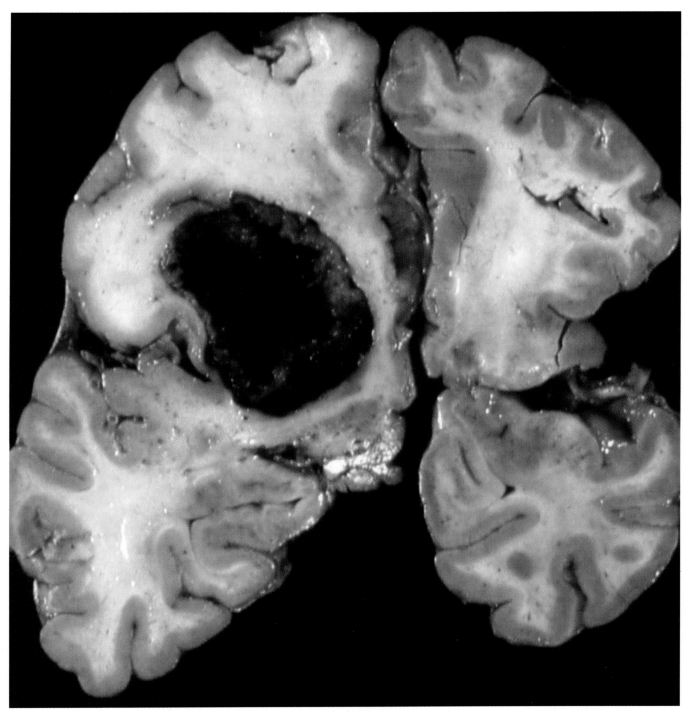

Figure 2.0-3: Metastatic carcinoma in the brain. Photo courtesy of Doug Miller, MD.

Benign tumors form when gene defects lead to a proliferation of cells that lack the capacity to aggressively invade normal tissue or metastasize to other sites. Sometimes benign tumors can undergo additional mutations and transform into malignant tumors. Table 2.0A lists some of the most common types of tumors and their cell of origin.

Most cancers arise in the skin or the lining of our internal organs, which are the parts of our body most exposed to carcinogens. Tissues such as muscle and bone, which have less exposure to carcinogens, are less likely to develop cancer.

The surface of our skin and the lining of our internal organs are made up of tissue called epithelium. Malignant tumors of epithelium are called carcinomas. Carcinomas are the most common type of cancer. Carcinomas usually resemble the type of epithelium they arise from. For example, the mouth is lined by squamous epithelium, and most cancers of the mouth are squamous cell carcinomas. In many sites, carcinomas are often preceded by an abnormal but benign precursor lesion such as dysplasia or hyperplasia. These abnormal proliferations sometimes last for years before an invasive carcinoma develops. Treatment at this stage can prevent cancer, and examples of precursor lesions will be discussed later in this chapter.

TABLE 2.0A
TUMORS BASED ON CELL TYPE

ORIGIN	BENIGN TUMOR	MALIGNANT TUMOR
glandular epithelium	adenoma	adenocarcinoma
squamous epithelium	squamous papilloma	squamous cell carcinoma
urothelium	urothelial papilloma	urothelial carcinoma
fat	lipoma	liposarcoma
fibrous tissue	fibroma	fibrosarcoma
blood vessels	hemangioma	angiosarcoma
smooth muscle	leiomyoma	leiomyosarcoma
skeletal muscle	rhabdomyoma	rhabdomyosarcoma
bone	osteoma	osteosarcoma
cartilage	chondroma	chondrosarcoma
melanocyte	melanocytic nevus	melanoma
nerves	neurofibroma	malignant peripheral nerve sheath tumor

Table 2.0B describes the leading sites of new cancer cases and the most common causes of deaths related to cancer in the United States in 2010 (2).

TABLE 2.0B
ESTIMATED 2010 UNITED STATES
NEW CANCER CASES AND DEATHS BY SITE (2)

SITE OF ORIGIN	NEW CASES	DEATHS
Lung	222,520	157,300
Colon/rectum	142,570	51,370
Breast	209,060	40,230
Prostate	217,730	32,050
Pancreas	43,140	36,800
Mouth/pharynx/larynx	49,260	11,480
Stomach/esophagus	37,640	25,070
Uterus	55,670	12,160
Skin (melanoma only)	68,130	8,700

Two terms used to describe cancers are the tumor's grade and stage. The grade is a measure of the tumor's differentiation based on what it looks like under the microscope. Well-differentiated tumors show differentiation similar to their cell of origin. For example, a well-differentiated squamous cell carcinoma resembles the normal squamous epithelium, which covers the skin and lines the mouth (Figs. 2.0-4, 2.0-5).

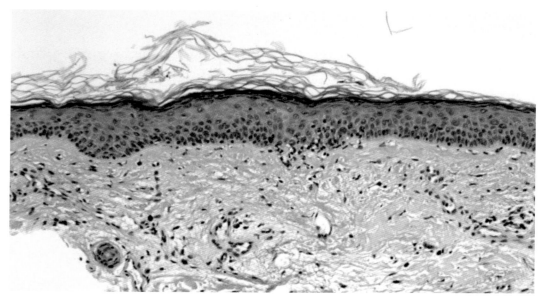

Figure 2.0-4: Normal squamous epithelium on the surface of the skin.

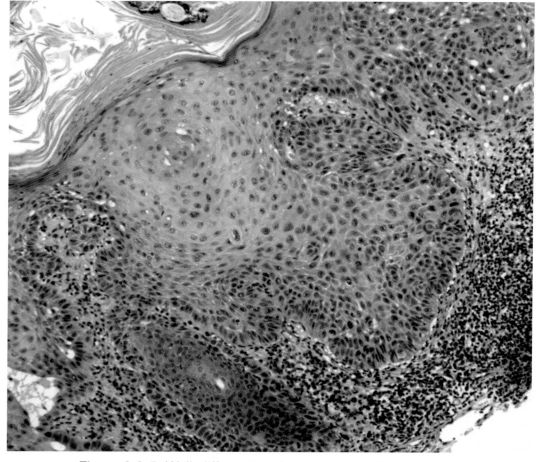

Figure 2.0-5: Well-differentiated squamous cell carcinoma.

It can be difficult to tell whether these tumors are malignant based on their appearance under the microscope. As cancers become more poorly differentiated, it is easier to tell whether they are malignant; however, it may be difficult to decipher the type of tumor. The moderately differentiated squamous cell carcinoma in Fig. 2.0-6 shows squamous differentiation as manifested by keratin production (the orange balls) similar to that which is produced in the normal squamous epithelium. However, the cells are more atypical and disorganized.

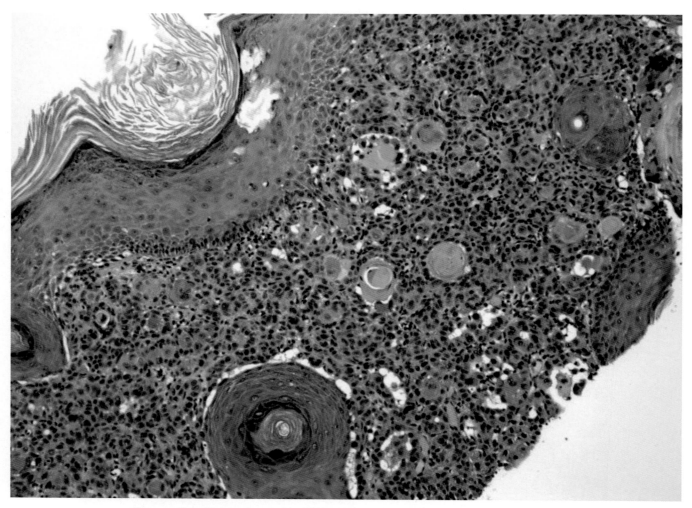

Figure 2.0-6: Moderately differentiated squamous cell carcinoma.

A poorly differentiated squamous cell carcinoma (Fig. 2.0-7) usually shows only focal areas resembling the squamous epithelium from which it arose. Poorly differentiated tumors are generally associated with a worse prognosis than well-differentiated tumors.

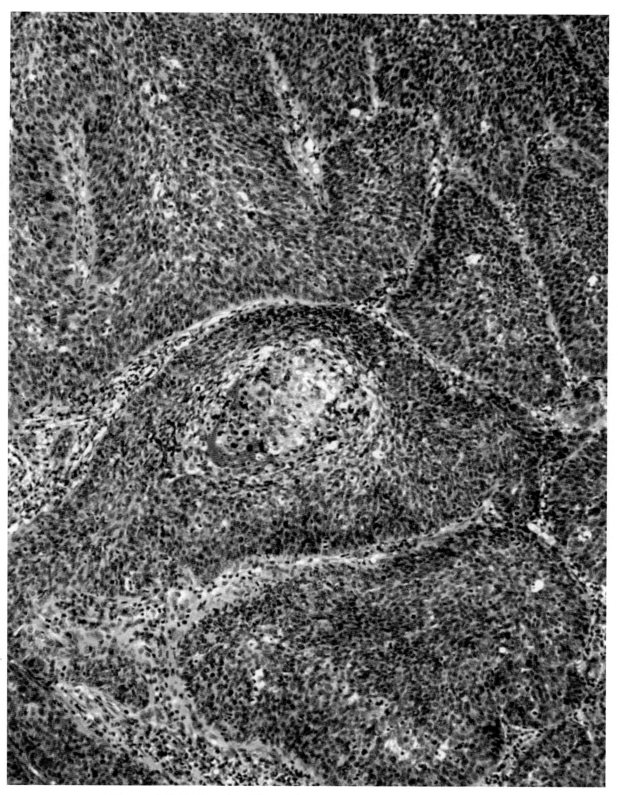

Figure 2.0-7: Poorly differentiated squamous cell carcinoma.

The stage of a tumor is a measure of how much the cancer has spread in the body. There are complex staging systems for each kind of cancer. In general, small cancers localized to their site of origin are stage 1. Large tumors or tumors with local metastases, such as adjacent lymph nodes, are generally stage 2 or 3. Tumors with metastatic disease affecting organs away from the primary site are usually stage 4. For most tumors, stage is a very powerful predictor of behavior; higher-stage tumors have a worse prognosis. It is very important to detect and treat cancer at an early stage. Neglected cancers can be devastating (Figs. 2.0-8 to 2.0-11).

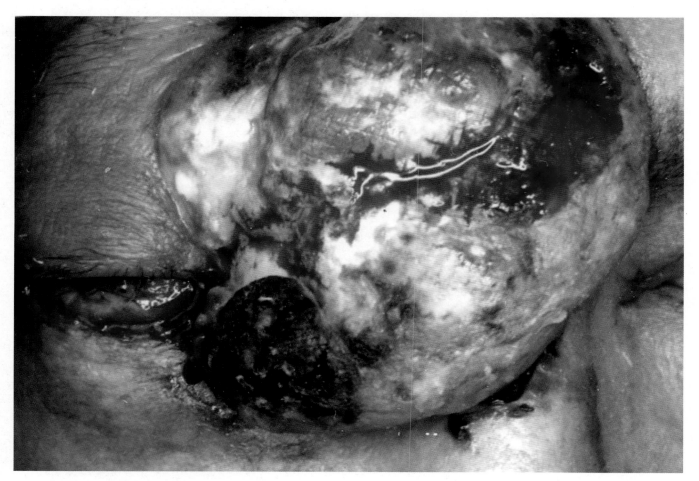

Figure 2.0-8: Advanced skin cancer with destruction of eye. Photo courtesy of Steve Westgate, MD.

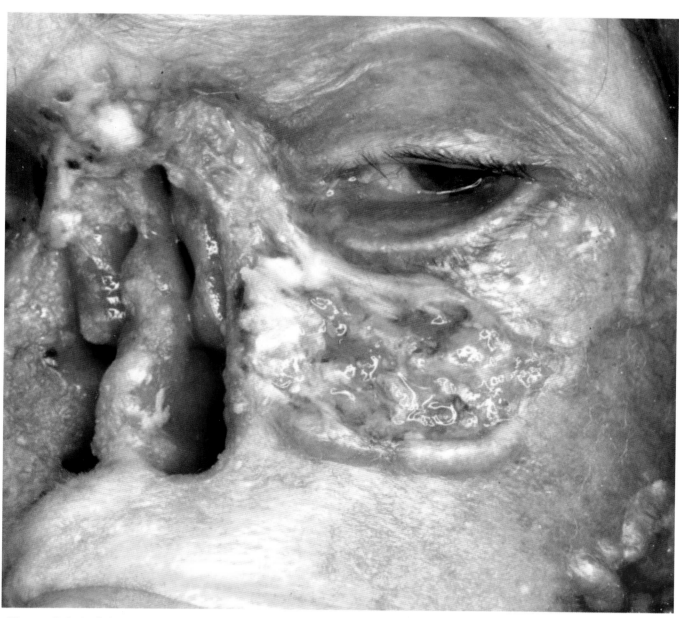

Figure 2.0-9: Advanced skin cancer with destruction of nose. Photo courtesy of Steve Westgate, MD.

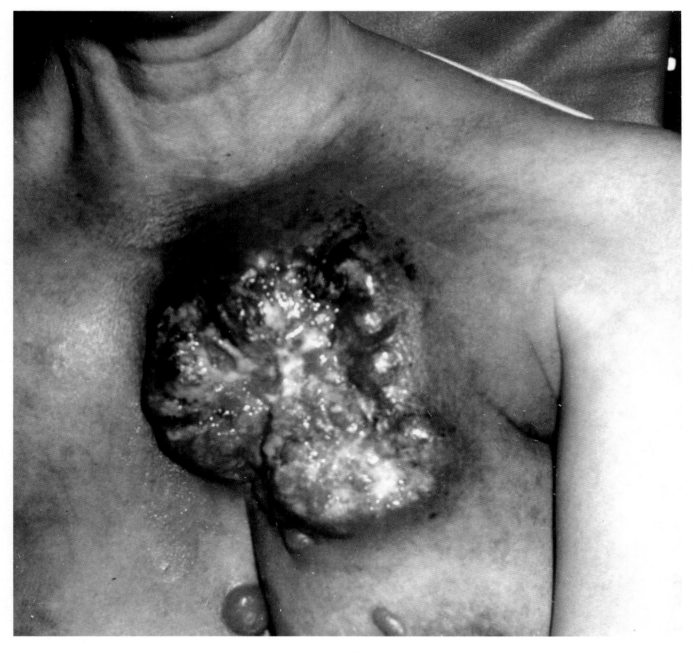

Figure 2.0-10: Advanced breast cancer. Photo courtesy of Steve Westgate, MD.

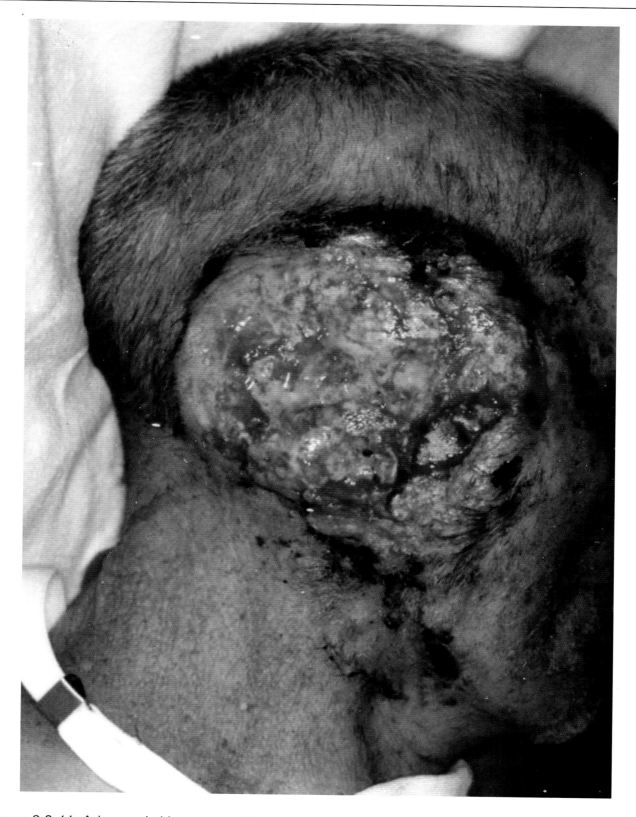

Figure 2.0-11: Advanced skin cancer with destruction of ear. Photo courtesy of Steve Westgate, MD.

PREVENTION

The American Cancer Society estimates that about one-third of the cancer deaths in the United States are caused by tobacco use (1). Another one-third are related to obesity, physical inactivity, and diet (1). Of the more than 1 million skin cancer cases seen each year in the United States, many could be prevented by avoiding excess sun exposure. Some cancers are related to infectious agents such as human papillomavirus (HPV), human immunodeficiency virus (HIV), Hepatitis B Virus (HBV), and Helicobacter pylori (H. pylori). Many of these can be prevented through behavioral changes such as avoiding IV drug abuse and high-risk sexual practices. Others can be prevented by vaccines or antibiotics (1). Cancer screening procedures such as pap smears, mammograms, and colonoscopies can find and eliminate precursor lesions and early cancers while they are still at a curable stage.

PERSONAL OBSERVATIONS
Cancer diagnosis is the most important job of a surgical pathologist. I have seen cancer affect every organ of the body. I have diagnosed cancer in patients of all age groups. I've listened to many tragic stories about how these tumors have destroyed lives. Please pay attention to the information in this chapter. It could prevent needless suffering for you and your loved ones.

RECOMMENDATIONS FOR DECREASING YOUR RISK OF CANCER
1. Don't smoke.
2. Maintain a healthy weight.
3. Exercise.
4. Eat a plant-based diet.
5. Avoid alcohol.
6. Avoid excessive sun exposure.
7. Don't engage in unsafe sexual practices.
8. Steer clear of IV drug abuse.
9. Follow cancer screening recommendations.

Detailed information about the most common cancers, their risk factors, and tips on prevention is outlined in the following sections.

REFERENCES:
1. American Cancer Society. "Cancer Facts & Figures 2011." Atlanta, GA: American Cancer Society, 2011.

2. American Cancer Society. "Cancer Facts & Figures 2010." Atlanta, GA: American Cancer Society, 2010.

2.1: LUNG CANCER

Worldwide, lung cancer kills more people than any other type. The incidence of lung cancer is closely related to the smoking rates of a population. In the United States, for example, lung cancer was rare before 1930, with approximately five cases per 100,000 people. Its prevalence increased as more people began smoking, peaking in 1984 with 102 cases per 100,000 people. As smoking rates have declined over the past thirty years, the incidence of lung cancer has also decreased. Currently there are about seventy-eight cases per 100,000 people (1). According to the National Cancer Institute, smoking causes 90 percent of the lung cancer deaths in men and 80 percent of the lung cancer deaths in women.

BACKGROUND INFORMATION

Bronchi are rigid tubular air spaces lined by epithelium with cilia, which beat like brooms to keep the airways clean (Fig. 2.1-1). These tubes deliver air to thin-walled air sacs called alveoli (Fig. 2.1-2), where the exchange of oxygen and carbon dioxide occurs during respiration.

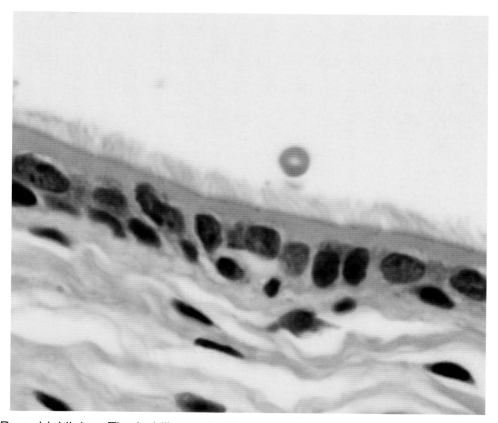

Figure 2.1-1: Bronchial lining. The hairlike projections are cilia, which beat and sweep the airway clean. The red circle is a red blood cell.

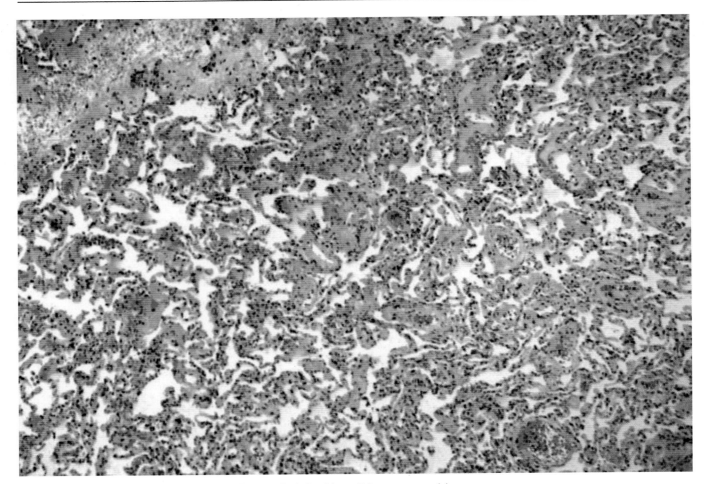

Figure 2.1-2: Alveoli in a normal lung.

PATHOLOGY

Most lung cancers arise from epithelium of the bronchi, which has the most exposure to the carcinogens in the air we breathe. The four most common types of lung cancer are squamous cell carcinoma, adenocarcinoma, small cell carcinoma, and large cell carcinoma (Figs. 2.1-3 to 2.1-8). Small cell carcinoma is a highly aggressive cancer that is usually metastatic at the time of diagnosis. It usually responds to chemotherapy, at least for a time. The other major types of lung carcinoma are less aggressive, but they are also less likely to respond to chemotherapy. Because of these features, lung cancer is often clinically grouped into small cell carcinomas and non–small cell carcinomas.

Lung cancer is a serious disease, with a combined five-year survival rate of only 16 percent. About half of the patients with early localized disease at the time of diagnosis survive. Unfortunately, lung cancer is usually advanced by the time it causes enough symptoms for patients to seek medical attention (1).

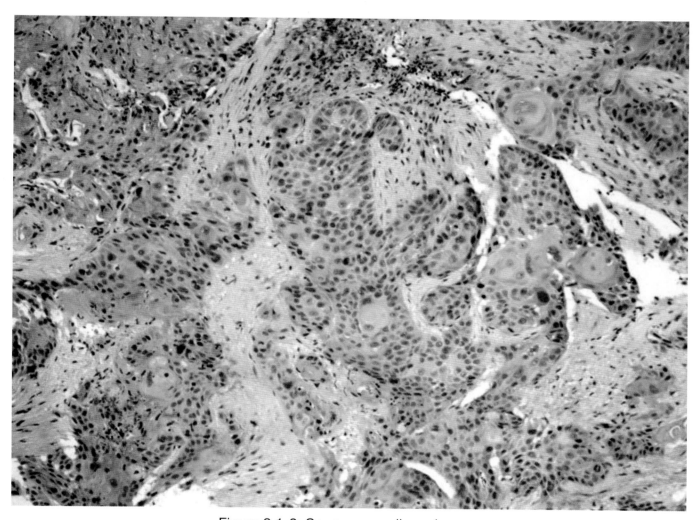

Figure 2.1-3: Squamous cell carcinoma.

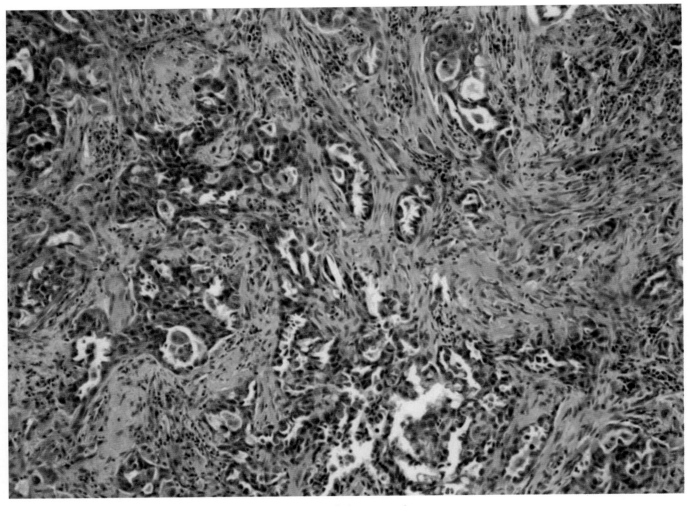

Figure 2.1-4: Adenocarcinoma.

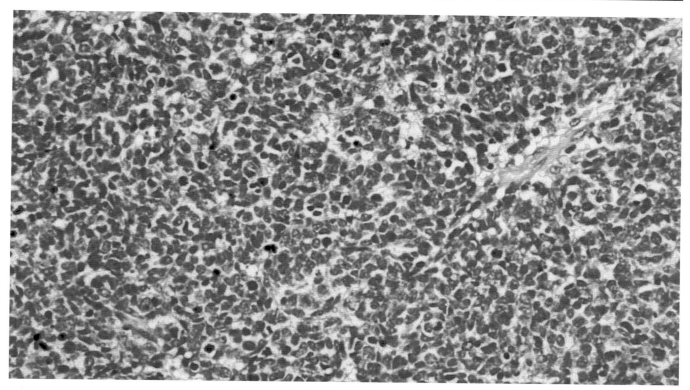

Figure 2.1-5: Small cell carcinoma.

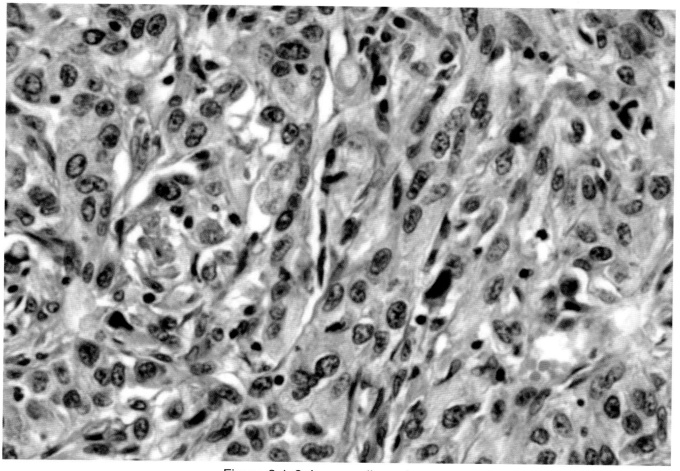

Figure 2.1-6: Large cell carcinoma.

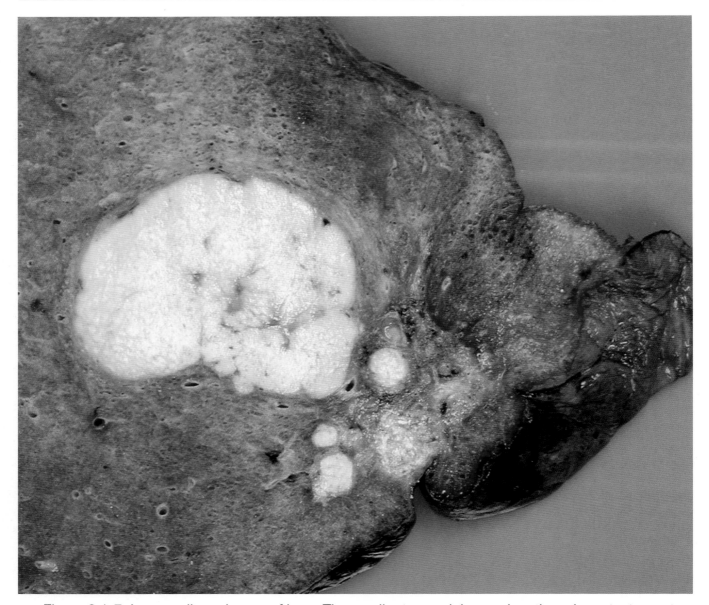

Figure 2.1-7: Large cell carcinoma of lung. The smaller tan nodules are lymph node metastases.

RISK FACTORS

Tobacco smoking: Eighty-seven percent of lung cancers occur in smokers (2). Compared with nonsmokers, heavy smokers—defined as those who smoke more than forty cigarettes per day for several years—have a sixty-fold greater risk of developing lung cancer (2). More than 1,200 substances have been found in cigarette smoke, many of which are carcinogens (2). These include both initiators (substances that directly damage DNA) as well as promoters (substances that encourage the proliferation of mutated cells).

Asbestos: A substance widely used in the insulation of buildings constructed between 1940 and 1989, asbestos acts as a carcinogen when inhaled. Its effects are additive to other factors such as smoking. For example, construction workers exposed to asbestos who do not smoke are five times more likely to develop lung cancer than the nonsmoking, non-asbestos-exposed population; exposed workers who do smoke are up to ninety times more likely to develop lung cancer (2).

Radiation: Radiation acts as a carcinogen through direct damage to DNA. An increased incidence of lung cancer has been seen among survivors of atomic bomb blasts as well as miners of uranium. Radon is a radioactive gas present in the air that comes from the decay of radioactive substances in the soil. While radon is detectable in nearly all air, it can reach high levels in some places, such as buildings with cracked foundations and poor ventilation. Some areas, such as the northern and Midwest portions of the United States, are especially likely to have elevated soil radon levels. Homes with poorly ventilated basements and cracked foundations may accumulate radon, resulting in significant radiation exposure for those who live inside. About one in fifteen homes in this country have elevated radon levels. The National Cancer Institute estimates that radon causes up to 10 percent of the lung cancer deaths in the US each year. Radon levels can easily and inexpensively be measured in your house. The Environmental Protection Agency maintains a free hotline (1-800-SOS-RADON) with information including regional radon testing agencies.

PERSONAL OBSERVATIONS

As I mentioned in the introduction, a common history submitted with biopsies of a lung cancer is that the patient was a longtime smoker but quit two weeks ago. The reason that this history is so common is that once a cancer starts causing signs and symptoms, many people have increased motivation to quit smoking. Unfortunately by the time a cancer gets a patient's attention, it has often reached a lethal stage. My goal in writing this chapter is to help people adopt a healthy lifestyle before they develop a deadly cancer.

Lung cancer is a terrible disease. It can reduce a healthy person to a skin-covered skeleton in only a few months. It is also one of the most preventable cancers. If you don't smoke, don't start. If you do smoke, quit. Have the radon levels in your home checked. Avoid asbestos exposure. Following these simple rules will help you avoid the vast majority of these tumors.

REFERENCES:

1. American Cancer Society. "Cancer Facts & Figures 2007." Atlanta, GA: American Cancer Society, 2007.

2. Husain AN, Kumar V. "The Lung." In *Robbins and Cotran Pathologic Basis of Disease*, 7th ed., edited by Kumar et al, 758. Philadelphia, PA: Elsevier Saunders, 2005.

2.2: COLORECTAL CANCER

Approximately 150,000 cases of colorectal cancer occur each year in the United States. These tumors kill over 50,000 US citizens per year, and equate to over 10 percent of all cancer-related deaths (1). Colorectal cancer occurs worldwide but varies greatly in incidence. The highest death rates are in the US, Australia, New Zealand, and Eastern Europe. Mexico, South America, and Africa have up to a ten-fold lower rate of colorectal cancer (2). When people from low-risk areas adopt a sedentary "Western lifestyle" with a diet high in meat, fat, and alcohol but low in fruits, vegetables, and fiber, their colon cancer risk increases to levels seen in the West. Fortunately, as the following indicates, the risk can significantly decrease with the implementation of lifestyle changes.

BACKGROUND INFORMATION

The large intestine, consisting of the colon and rectum, has a simple job. It stores fecal material before elimination and absorbs water and electrolytes. It is a muscular tube lined by mucosa and is made up of glandular epithelium (Fig. 2.2-1). Because fecal material is in contact with the lining of the large intestine longer than other parts of the GI tract, the large intestinal mucosa has the potential to be in contact with carcinogens longer than other areas of the bowel.

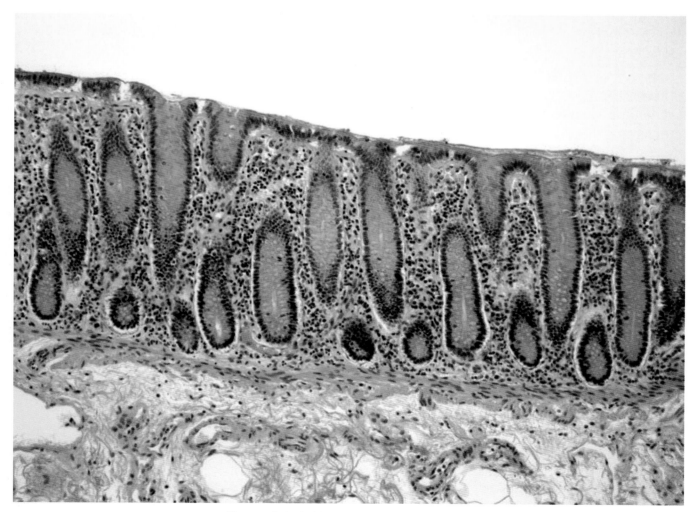

Figure 2.2-1: Normal colonic mucosa.

PATHOLOGY

Over 90 percent of the cancers of the large intestine are adenocarcinomas. Most colorectal adenocarcinomas are thought to develop in preexisting benign glandular tumors called adenomas. Initial DNA mutations lead to the formation of the benign adenomas, and subsequent additional mutations cause adenocarcinoma to develop in the adenomas (Figs. 2.2-2 to 2.2-6). Adenomas are often small and may exist for years before cancer develops in them. The presence of this adenoma-carcinoma sequence in colon cancer provides an opportunity to find and treat tumors before they develop into lethal cancers. Removal of colonic adenomas and even noninvasive adenocarcinomas is associated with nearly a 100 percent cure rate. On the other hand, advanced colon cancer with metastatic spread to other organs (Fig. 2.2-6) has a five-year survival rate of only 10 percent.

Fortunately, there is a procedure called screening colonoscopy where doctors can find and remove colon tumors at a very early stage. During this procedure, a doctor examines the colon with a small flexible scope to find any existing tumors. Most small tumors can be removed as part of this procedure. A screening colonoscopy is recommended for anyone fifty years or older, and earlier in patients with a family history of colon cancer or other increased risk factors, such as those outlined later in this chapter. Unfortunately, the rate of screening is low, and many patients are diagnosed with colon cancer after the disease has already progressed.

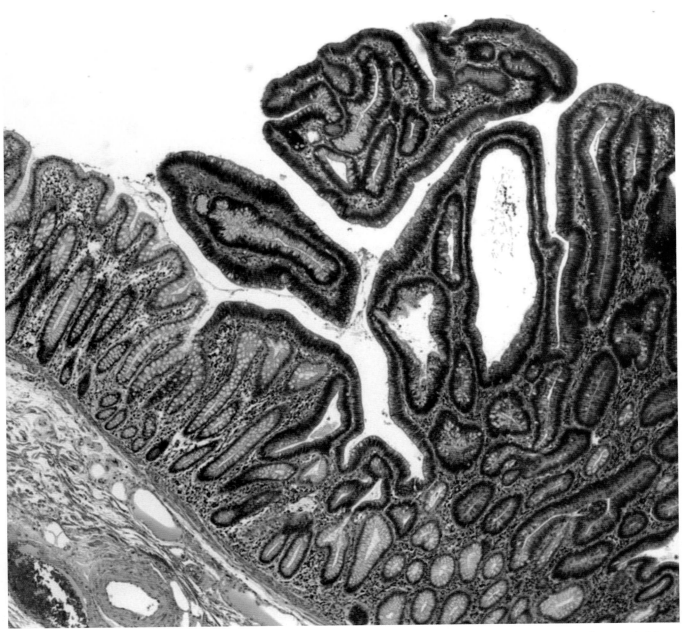

Figure 2.2-2: Tubulovillous adenoma (center and right) next to normal colonic mucosa (upper left).

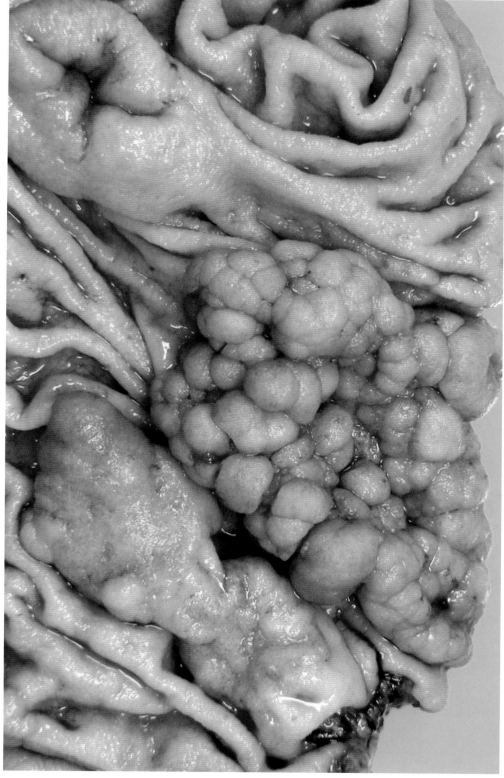

Figure 2.2-3: Adenocarinoma (smooth pink) arising in an adenoma (multinodular tan).

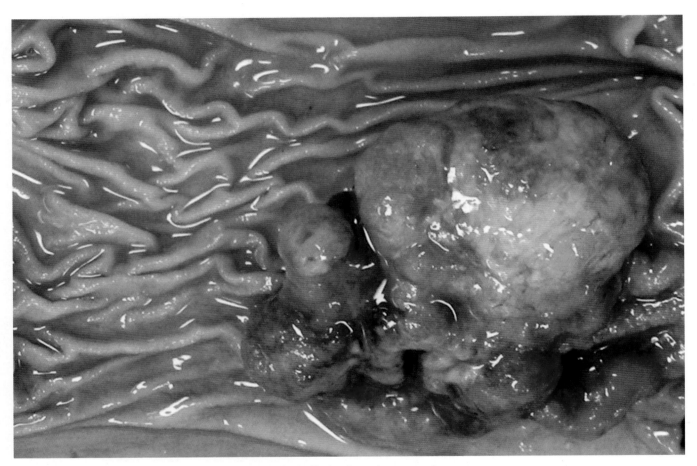

Figure 2.2-4: Colonic adenocarcinoma.

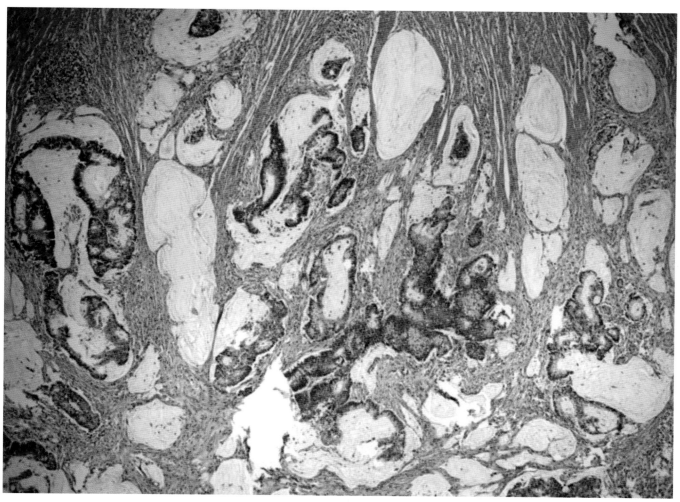

Figure 2.2-5: Colonic adenocarcinoma.

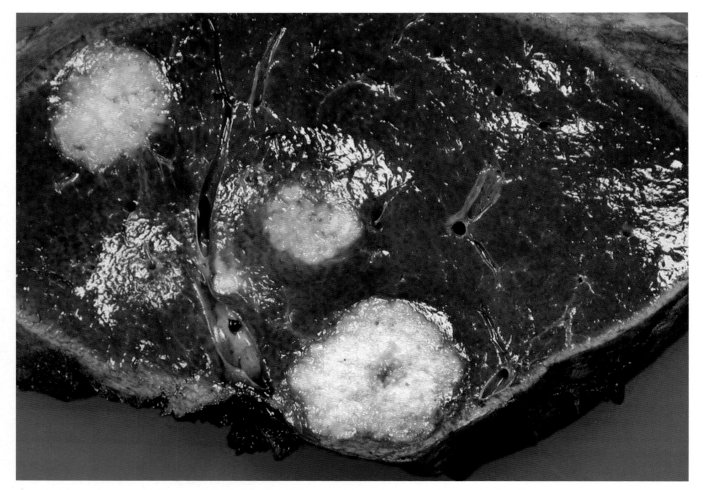

Figure 2.2-6: Metastatic colonic adenocarcinoma in the liver.

RISK FACTORS

Some factors associated with an increased risk of colon cancer cannot be prevented. These include age (90 percent of colon cancers occur in patients fifty years and older), history of previous colonic adenomas or adenocarcinoma, inflammatory bowel disease, and a family history of colon cancer (3). Rare inherited syndromes associated with a high incidence of colonic adenomas and adenocarcinomas include familial adenomatous polyposis, hereditary nonpolyposis colon cancer, Turcot syndrome, and Peutz-Jeghers syndrome (3). African Americans and Jews of Eastern European descent (known as Ashkenazi Jews) also have an increased risk of developing the disease (3).

Fortunately, however, many of the risk factors associated with colon cancer can be prevented with a change in lifestyle. For example, eating red meat is associated with an increased risk of colon cancer, whereas diets rich in fruits and vegetables lower the risk of developing the disease. Other factors associated with increased risk include physical inactivity, obesity, type 2 diabetes, smoking, and alcohol use (3).

Studies have shown that aspirin and other anti-inflammatory drugs are associated with a decreased incidence of both colonic adenomas and colonic cancers. How these drugs help protect against colon cancer is not fully understood. However, it is thought that these agents inhibit the production of substances called prostaglandins, which may be involved in the metabolism of tumor cells (2). A calcium-rich diet and vitamin D supplements may also reduce the risk of colon cancer (4, 5). Details on how these nutrients protect against colon cancer are outlined in chapter 13.

In short, you can markedly decrease your risk of colon cancer through lifestyle adjustments and cancer screening. Cancer screening should begin at age fifty or earlier if you have increased risk factors such as a family history of colon cancer. Some people avoid getting a colonoscopy because they are embarrassed or fear the procedure. However, I can tell you from experience that it is not that bad. The bowel prep is a bit unpleasant because it involves a short fast from solid food and several hours of diarrhea. The actual procedure is done in a private manner and is virtually pain free if done by a competent physician. One thing is for sure: a screening colonoscopy is a piece of cake compared to having colon cancer!

PERSONAL OBSERVATIONS

I used to know a difficult man who boasted once that he never saw a doctor, never took any medications or supplements, and avoided sun exposure. As a result he never had a screening colonoscopy and was almost certainly vitamin D deficient, as he was also inactive, overweight, and ate a typical meat-rich Western diet. Soon after we spoke, I diagnosed adenocarcinoma on his colon biopsy. He died from his cancer within two years. Colon cancer is largely preventable but can be devastating if you don't take precautions. Don't let this happen to you!

REFERENCES:

1. American Cancer Society. "Cancer Facts & Figures 2007." Atlanta, GA: American Cancer Society, 2007.

2. Liu C, Crawford JM. "The Gastrointestinal Tract." In *Robbins and Cotran Pathologic Basis of Disease*, 7th ed., edited by Kumar et al, 864–65. Philadelphia, PA: Elsevier Saunders, 2005.

3. American Cancer Society. "What Are the Risk Factors for Colorectal Cancer?" Atlanta, GA: American Cancer Society, 2009.

4. American Cancer Society. "Calcium May Reduce Risk of Colon Cancer." Atlanta, GA: American Cancer Society, 2003.

5. Holick MF. "Vitamin D Deficiency." *New England Journal of Medicine* 357 (2007): 266–81.

2.3: BREAST CANCER

Breast cancer is the most frequently diagnosed cancer in women. A woman who lives to age ninety has a one-in-eight chance of developing the disease (1). In the United States alone, about 178,000 women are diagnosed and over 40,000 women die of breast cancer each year (2). Early detection saves lives and increases treatment options. Currently, the five-year survival rate for small, localized breast cancers is 98 percent (2). If distant metastases are present, the five-year survival rate drops to 26 percent (2). Breast cancer screening, including self-examinations, clinical breast exams, and mammograms (recommended annually after age forty) are helpful in detecting tumors at an early and potentially curable stage. It is never a good idea to neglect or ignore any type of cancer. It will only get worse (Fig. 2.3-1).

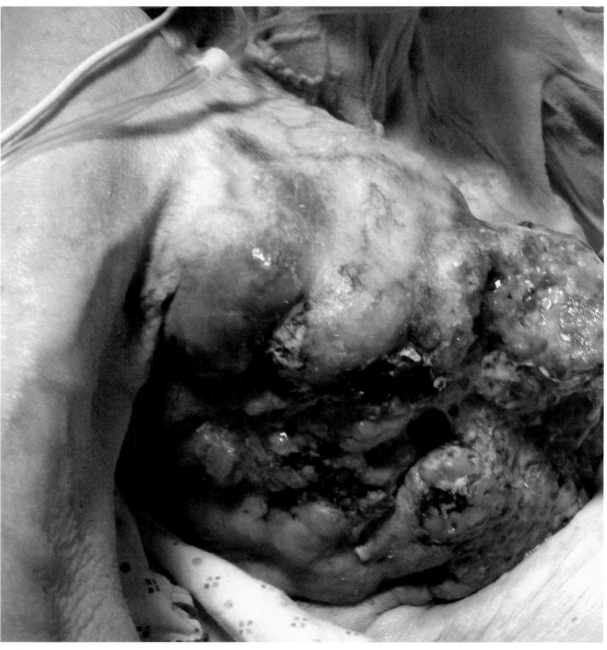

Figure 2.3-1: Advanced neglected breast cancer. Photo courtesy of Eugene Shively, MD.

BACKGROUND INFORMATION

The human female breast has six to ten major ducts emptying into the nipple. The large ducts branch into terminal duct lobular units where the milk is produced (Figs. 2.3-2, 2.3-3). The terminal duct lobular unit is also the site where most cancers, and a potentially precancerous condition called fibrocystic changes, arise.

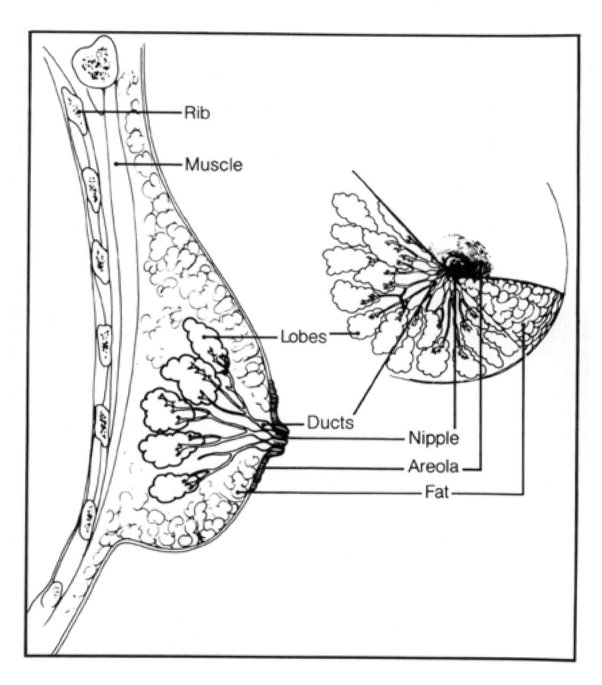

Figure 2.3-2: Structure of normal breast. Image courtesy of Susan Spangler, National Cancer Institute.

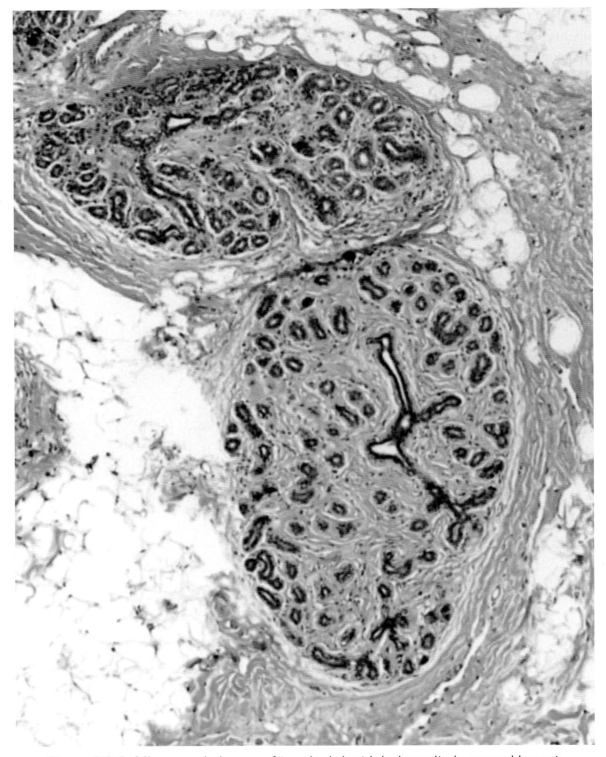

Figure 2.3-3: Microscopic image of terminal duct lobular units in normal breast.

PATHOLOGY

Over time, most women develop fibrocystic changes in the breast. Nonproliferative changes, such as cysts, are not associated with an increased risk of breast cancer. However, some types of fibrocystic changes have proliferation of the glandular cells lining the ducts and lobules. When this is present, the patient has an increased risk of developing breast cancer. Pathologists group fibrocystic change into categories of no increased risk, slight increased risk (1.5 to 2 times increased risk), or moderate increased risk (4 to 5 times increased risk) based on the changes seen under the microscope.

Most breast cancers arise from the lining of the ducts and lobules and are types of adenocarcinoma. The term "carcinoma in situ" is used to describe breast cancers that are still limited to the ducts and lobules. When the tumor breaks out of the normal terminal duct lobular unit and invades the adjacent breast tissue, it is an invasive carcinoma. In-situ and invasive carcinomas are classified according to their resemblance to normal structures (Figs. 2.3-4 to 2.3-7). The two major types of in-situ carcinoma are ductal carcinoma in situ and lobular carcinoma in situ.

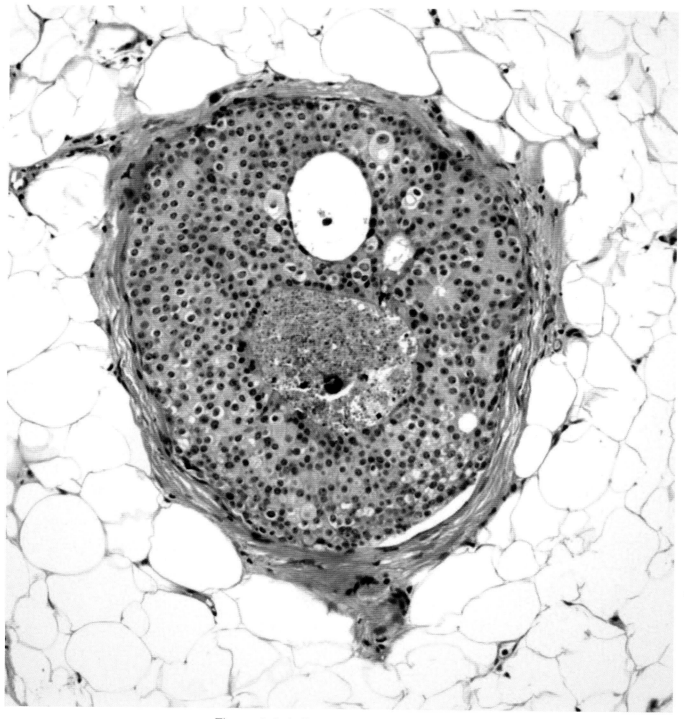

Figure 2.3-4: Ductal carcinoma in situ.

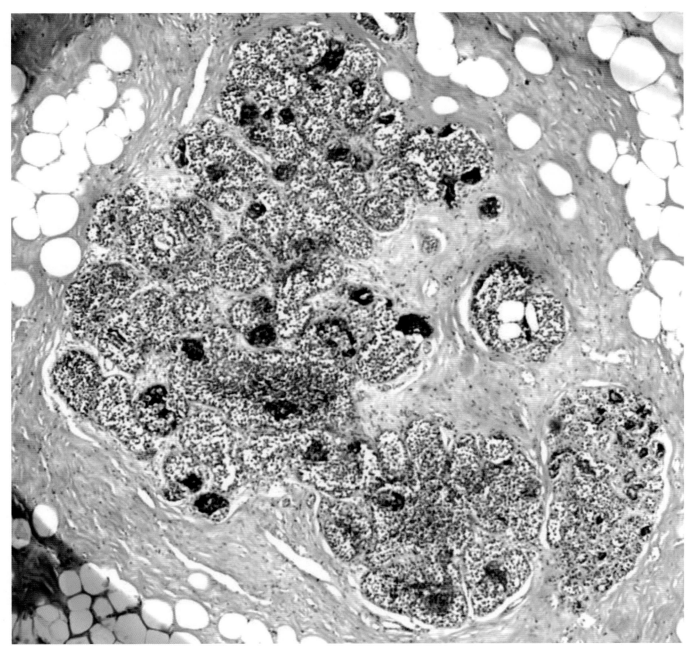

Figure 2.3-5: Lobular carcinoma in situ.

The most common invasive carcinoma is invasive ductal carcinoma (or invasive carcinoma of no special type).

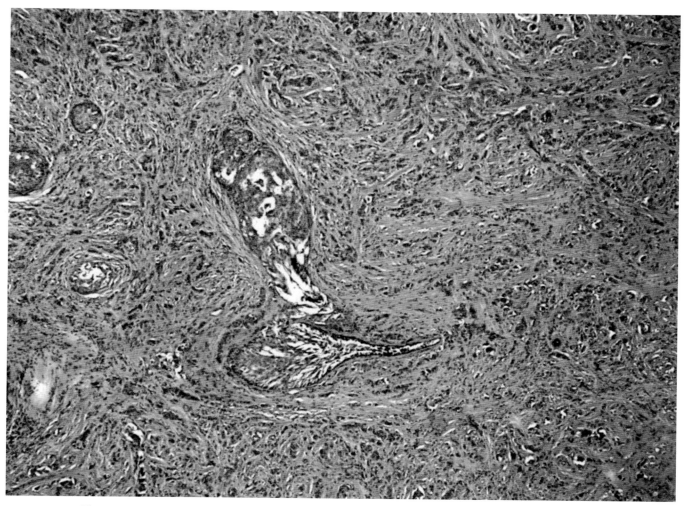

Figure 2.3-6: Ductal carcinoma in situ surrounded by invasive ductal carcinoma.

The second-most-common type of invasive carcinoma is invasive lobular carcinoma.

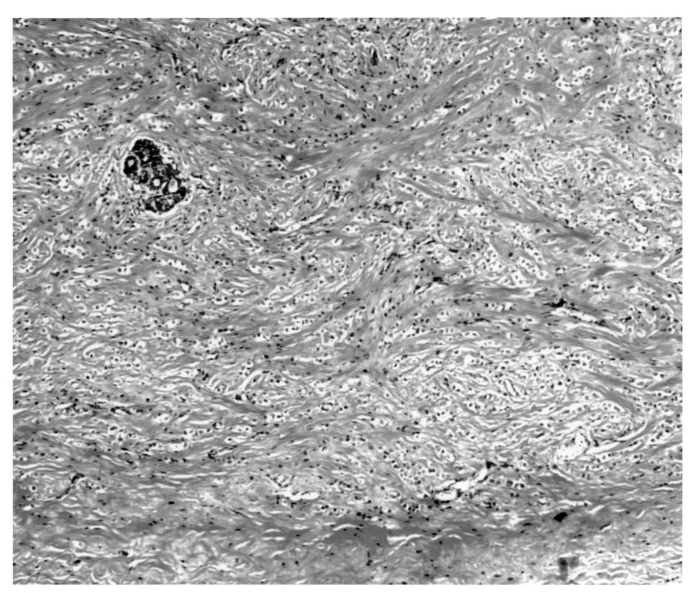

Figure 2.3-7: Invasive lobular carcinoma.

Ductal carcinoma in situ is often associated with calcifications and can often be detected by mammogram before invasion occurs. Invasive carcinomas show irregular armlike extensions into the surrounding stroma. It is thought that the term "cancer" (which is the Latin word for "crab") was first used to describe the crablike infiltrative growth of invasive ductal carcinoma (Fig. 2.3-8).

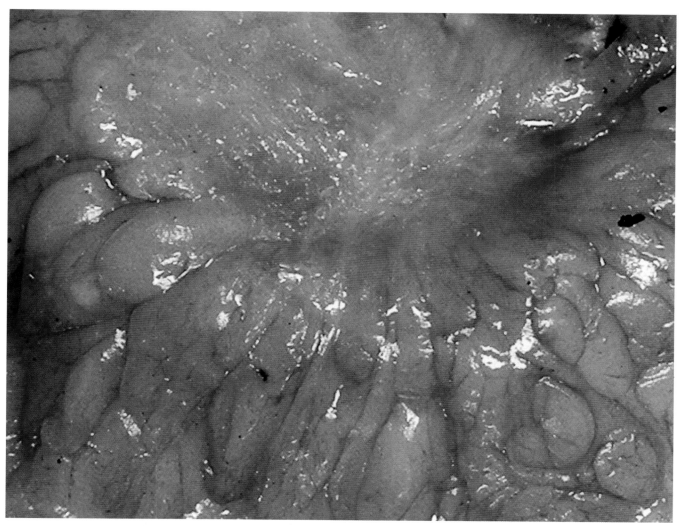

Figure 2.3-8: Invasive ductal carcinoma of breast. Note irregular fingerlike extensions of the tan tumor within yellow fatty stroma.

In-situ carcinoma of the breast can extend up the major ducts into nipple skin, resulting in an oozing, scaling crust. This condition is called Paget's disease, after Sir James Paget, who described the condition back in 1874 (3) (Fig. 2.3-9).

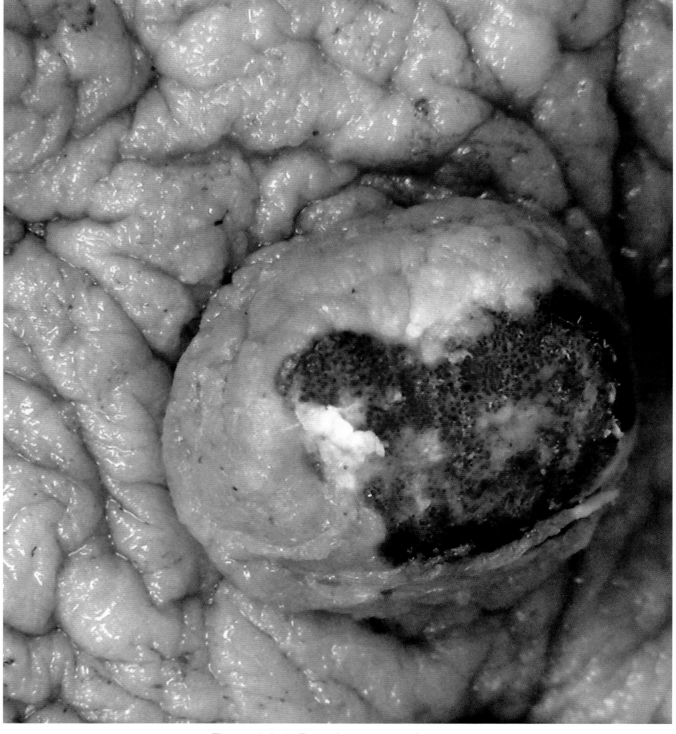

Figure 2.3-9: Paget's disease of nipple.

RISK FACTORS

Gender: While breast cancer can occur in men, it is about 100 times more common in women (1).

Age: The chances of developing breast cancer increase with age. It is rare before age twenty-five, and most cases occur after age fifty (1).

Family history: If you have a first-degree relative (mother, sister, or daughter) who was diagnosed with breast cancer before age fifty, you have an increased risk as well. Some families have an inherited mutation in genes called breast cancer 1 (BRCA1) or breast cancer 2 (BRCA2), which predisposes women to breast and ovarian cancers (1).

Early onset of menstrual cycles/late menopause: Early or prolonged exposure of breast tissue to estrogen (in other words, if you have your first period before age twelve or experience menopause beyond age fifty-five) are associated with an increased risk of breast cancer (1, 2).

Age of first pregnancy: Women who have their first full-term pregnancy before age twenty have half the risk of developing breast cancer as women who have never been pregnant or have become pregnant after age thirty-five. It is thought that pregnancy results in full maturation of breast lining cells, which may protect them from developing genetic mutations leading to cancer (1).

Hormone therapy: Postmenopausal estrogen replacement increases the risk of breast cancer 1.2- to 1.7-fold. Because replacing estrogen alone increases the risk of endometrial cancer, some doctors prescribe both estrogen and progesterone. While adding progesterone eliminates the increased risk for endometrial cancer, it increases the risk for breast cancer more than using only estrogen. Oral contraceptives in premenopausal women do not seem to significantly affect breast cancer risk (1).

Geographic influence: Breast cancer rates are four to seven times higher in the United States and Europe than in developing countries. The risk of breast cancer increases for immigrants to the United States.

Scientists are investigating whether the following modifiable risk factors are possible causes behind these findings (1):

Diet: While some studies have shown that a plant-based diet decreases the risk of breast cancer, this finding has not been confirmed (1). Vitamin D supplementation may decrease breast cancer risk up to 50 percent (4). Alcohol use, on the other hand, is associated with an increased risk (1, 2, 5).

Obesity: Postmenopausal obese women have an increased risk for breast cancer, potentially as a result of the estrogen produced in fatty tissue (1).

Exercise: Different studies have shown that thirty to sixty minutes of moderate or vigorous exercise per day reduces your breast cancer risk between 20 to 80 percent (6). An example of moderate exercise is walking for pleasure.

Breastfeeding: Breastfeeding is associated with reduced breast cancer risk; the longer women breastfeed, the greater the reduction in risk (1).

PERSONAL OBSERVATIONS

One of the saddest stories I've encountered as a surgical pathologist involved a twenty-seven-year-old woman who came to our hospital with advanced breast cancer. She had seen a physician in another town two years prior for a breast lump, but had been told not to worry about it since she was only twenty-five. While most breast lumps in young people are benign, cancer can happen at any age. Practice breast cancer screening and pursue the diagnosis of any suspicious findings.

REFERENCES:

1. Lester SC. "The Breast." In *Robbins and Cotran Pathologic Basis of Disease*, 8th ed., edited by Kumar et al, 1065–95. Philadelphia, PA: Elsevier Saunders, 2010.

2. American Cancer Society. "Cancer Facts & Figures 2007." Atlanta, GA: American Cancer Society, 2007.

3. Paget J. "On Disease of the Mammary Areola Preceding Cancer of the Mammary Gland." *St. Bartholomew's Hospital Reports* 10 (1874): 87–89.

4. Holick MF. "Vitamin D Deficiency." *New England Journal of Medicine* 357 (2007): 266–81.

5. Allen et al. "Moderate Alcohol Intake and Cancer Incidence in Women." *Journal of the National Cancer Institute* 101 (2009): 296–305.

6. National Cancer Institute. "Physical Activity and Cancer." Rockville, MD: NCI. Last reviewed July 22, 2009. http://www.cancer.gov/cancertopics/factsheet/prevention/physicalactivity.

2.4: PROSTATE CANCER

Prostate cancer is the most common form of cancer, and the second leading cause of cancer death in US males (1). In the United States, about 240,000 new cases of prostate cancer are diagnosed and about 34,000 men die of the disease each year. Prostate cancer is very common in older men. Autopsy studies of men dying from other causes have shown that about 70 percent of men older than age seventy have small prostate cancers (1).

It is not completely understood why some prostate cancers remain stable and others progress to cause life-threatening disease. Possible reasons for disease progression will be discussed later in the *pathology* section. Most small prostate cancers discovered incidentally when prostate tissue is removed for other causes do not progress to cause significant disease. These are called latent cancers. Prostate cancers that have progressed enough to come to the attention of doctors taking care of the patient are more likely to cause significant problems. These are called clinically evident cancers.

There are marked national and racial differences in the incidence of clinically evident prostate cancer. These cancers are rare in Asia but common in the United States, particularly among African Americans.

TABLE 2.4A
PEAK INCIDENCE OF CLINICALLY EVIDENT PROSTATIC CARCINOMA (CASES PER 100,000 POPULATION) (1, 2)

- Chinese: 1
- Japanese: 4
- US white males: 238
- US black males: 343

BACKGROUND INFORMATION

The prostate is a walnut-sized organ that sits beneath the bladder and encircles the urethra in men. Its secretions contribute to semen. It is made up of glands, which are maintained by male hormones such as testosterone and dihydrotestosterone. With age, almost all men develop prostatic nodular hyperplasia (also known as benign prostatic hypertrophy, or BPH). Enlargement of the prostate due to hyperplasia or cancer can obstruct the urethra, leading to urinary retention in the bladder (Fig. 2.4-1).

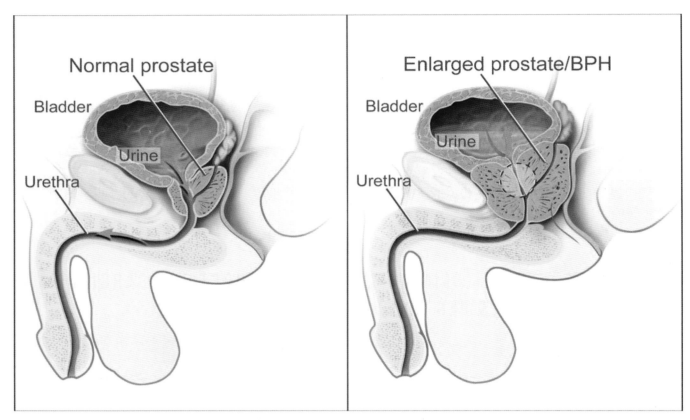

Figure 2.4-1: Normal and enlarged prostate.
Image courtesy of Alan Hoofring, National Cancer Institute.

PATHOLOGY

Prostate cancers are some of the most difficult tumors to see with the naked eye. They are usually in the peripheral portions of the gland and often are only evident by a firm yellow area (Fig. 2.4-2).

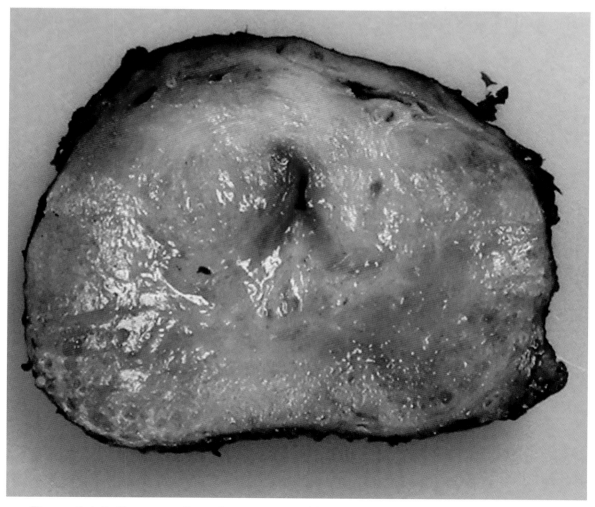

Figure 2.4-2: Cross section of a prostate with cancer (yellow area, bottom center). The red circle in the upper center of the photo is the urethra.

Most prostate cancers are adenocarcinomas (Fig. 2.4-3).

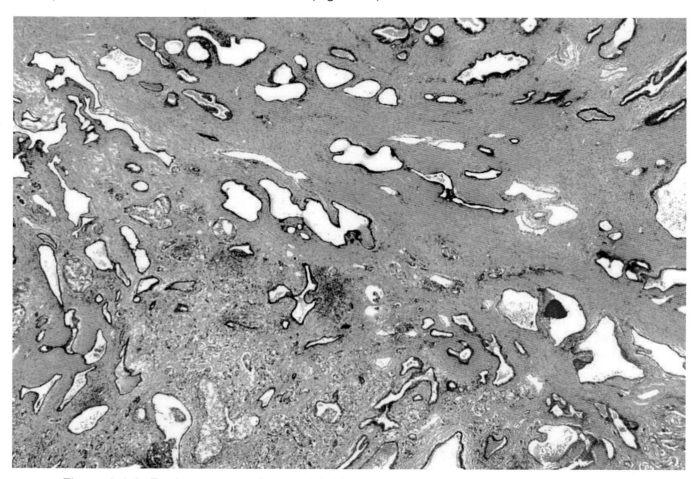

Figure 2.4-3: Benign prostate (upper right) being invaded by prostate cancer (lower left).

The most common grading system used for prostate cancer is the Gleason system, which groups prostatic adenocarcinomas into five types of patterns. Latent cancers can show any pattern of disease, while clinically evident cancers usually show only patterns 3, 4, or 5 (Figs. 2.4-4 to 2.4-6).

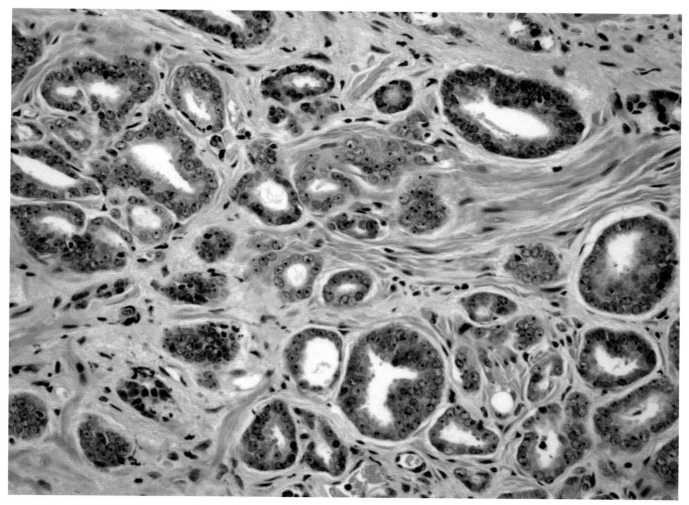

Figure 2.4-4: Gleason pattern 3, prostatic adenocarcinoma (infiltrative single separate glands).

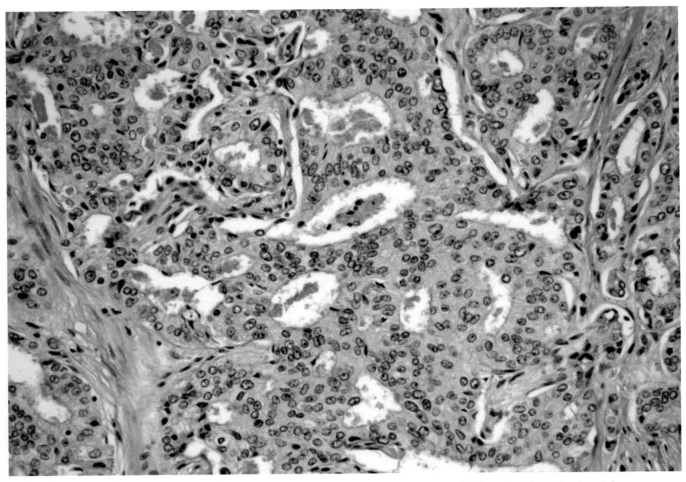

Figure 2.4-5: Gleason pattern 4, prostatic adenocarcinoma (infiltrative fused glands).

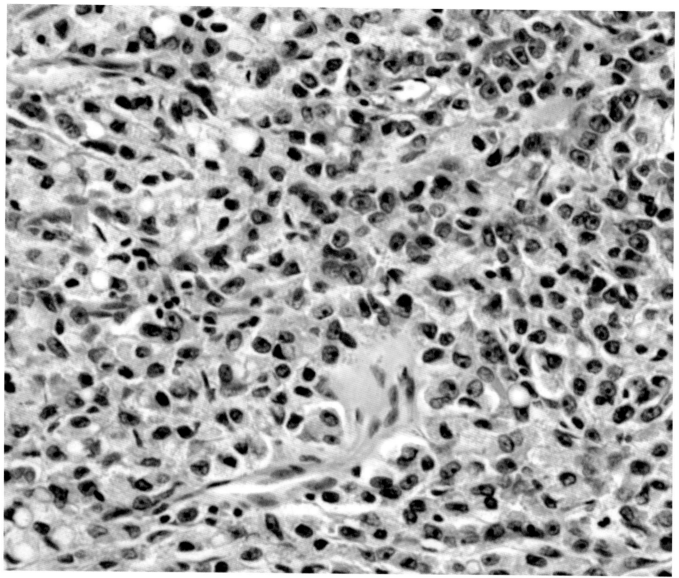

Figure 2.4-6: Gleason pattern 5, prostatic adenocarcinoma (near-solid/sheetlike architecture).

The two predominant patterns are added together to give a Gleason pattern score. If the tumor only has one pattern, that pattern is doubled to obtain the pattern score.

For example, if most of the tumor looks like pattern 3, but some looks like pattern 4, the Gleason score would be 7 (3 + 4). If the tumor all looks like pattern 5, the score would be 10 (5 + 5). Gleason scores are helpful in predicting behavior. Patients with a score of 4 or less almost never develop the aggressive form of the disease, while most patients with scores of 8 or higher are not likely to survive.

The stage of the disease also has a marked impact on the prognosis. Small latent cancers found incidentally in prostate tissue removed for nodular hyperplasia or other causes are associated with an excellent prognosis, while tumors with metastatic disease are usually fatal. Autopsy studies have found that these latent carcinomas are common in older men of both high-risk and low-risk populations. For example, Japanese and Caucasian Americans have about the same incidence of these latent tumors (1). It is likely that initial cellular mutations give rise to latent adenocarcinomas, and additional genetic or environmental factors may be required for these tumors to become aggressive enough to be clinically important (1).

An example of genetic factors involved in the progression of prostate cancer may be the relative sensitivity of prostatic cells to male hormones called androgens. Androgens stimulate prostate cells and are important in the development of prostate cancer. Studies have shown that prostate cells from men of different races have different androgen sensitivities: Asians have the lowest androgen sensitivity, US whites have intermediate sensitivity, and African Americans have the highest sensitivity (1). This may partially account for the varied progression of prostate cancers within these populations.

Environmental factors such as diet may also play a role in the progression of latent cancers into clinically important tumors. Notably, clinically detectable prostate cancer rates increase in Asians who immigrate to the United States.

Depending on the clinical findings and patient preference, current treatment for prostate cancer includes surgery, radiation therapy, and hormonal manipulations. Treatment is quite effective, with an overall ten-year survival rate of 93 percent and a fifteen-year survival rate of 77 percent (2). However, prostate cancers accompanied by metastatic disease are almost always fatal (1).

RISK FACTORS

Age, ethnicity, and family history of the disease are the established risk factors for prostate cancer. Obesity, smoking, and diets high in saturated fat may also contribute to the development of clinically significant disease (2, 6). Dietary products that may prevent, inhibit, or delay progression include soy products, vitamin D, lycopene, and selenium (3). Tomatoes, watermelon, and bell peppers are rich in lycopene. Good sources of selenium include Brazil nuts, grains, and fish.

Vitamin D may be an especially important determinant of prostate cancer risk, and 1 billion people worldwide get an insufficient amount (4). Prostate tissues have vitamin D receptors, and men with low blood levels of vitamin D have a 30 to 50 percent increased risk of prostate cancer (4). Dark-skinned people absorb less vitamin D from sun exposure than lighter-skinned individuals do, and a recent study found that 61 percent of African American men have a vitamin D deficiency (5). This deficiency may contribute to the high incidence of prostate cancer found in this population.

PERSONAL OBSERVATIONS

I have diagnosed hundreds of prostate cancers and seen the pain on the face of prostate cancer patients. It is a very common and potentially fatal disease. Fortunately, your risk can be minimized by not smoking, eating a plant-based diet, taking vitamin D supplements, and avoiding obesity.

REFERENCES:

1. Epstein JI. "The Lower Urinary Tract and Male Genital System." *Robbins and Cotran Pathologic Basis of Disease*, 7th ed., edited by Kumar et al, 1050–56. Philadelphia, PA: Elsevier Saunders, 2005.

2. American Cancer Society. "Cancer Facts & Figures 2007." Atlanta, GA: American Cancer Society, 2007.

3. Mazhar D, Waxman J. "Diet and Prostate Cancer." *British Journal of Urology International* 93, no. 7 (2004): 919–22.

4. Holick MF. "Vitamin D Deficiency." *New England Journal of Medicine* 357 (2007): 266–81.

5. Tseng et al. "Prevalence and Correlates of Vitamin D Status in African American Men." *BMC Public Health* 9 (2009): 191.

6. Kenfield et al. "Smoking and Prostate Cancer Survival and Recurrence." *Journal of the American Medical Association* 305 (2011): 2548–55.

2.5: PANCREATIC CANCER

Pancreatic cancer is the fourth leading cause of cancer-related death in the United States, preceded only by lung, colon, and breast cancers. It kills about 33,000 US citizens each year, and has one of the worst prognoses of all cancer types, with a five-year survival rate of less than 5 percent (1, 2).

BACKGROUND INFORMATION
Located beneath the stomach, the pancreas measures approximately 20 centimeters in length and weighs about 90 grams (Fig. 2.5-1).

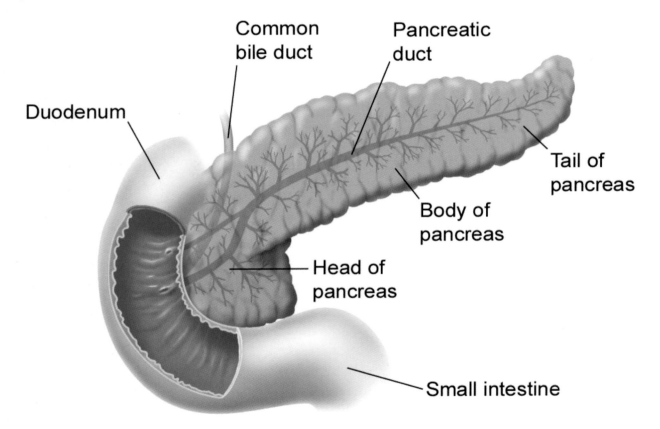

National Cancer Institute

Figure 2.5-1: Anatomy of the pancreas. Figure courtesy of Don Bliss, National Cancer Institute.

The pancreas has two major functions:
1. It produces enzymes that help us digest our food.
2. It produces hormones such as insulin, which helps us regulate blood sugar levels.

The digestive enzymes are delivered to the intestine through pancreatic ducts. The hormones are released directly into the blood.

PATHOLOGY
While there are many types of pancreatic tumors, most pancreatic cancers are adenocarcinomas, which

arise from the pancreatic ducts. These ductal adenocarcinomas fall under the more general term of "pancreatic cancer."

Pancreatic carcinomas often do not cause symptoms until they have either plugged up the main pancreatic duct, causing obstructive jaundice, or invaded adjacent nerves, causing pain (Fig. 2.5-2).

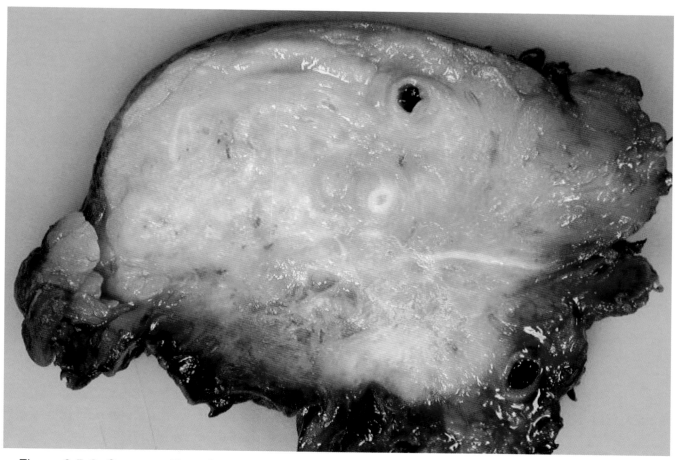

Figure 2.5-2: Cross section of a pancreatic adenocarcinoma. Note extension of the tan tumor into surrounding yellow fat.

Most cases at the time of diagnosis have already progressed to the point that they cannot be surgically removed (Fig. 2.5-3).

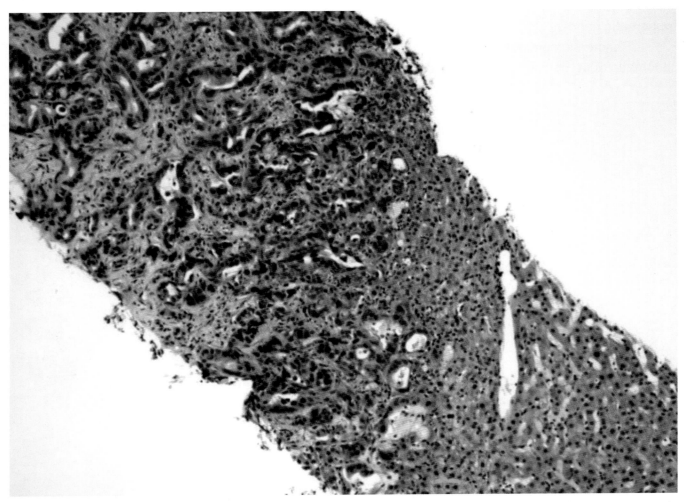

Figure 2.5-3: Liver biopsy showing metastatic pancreatic adenocarcinoma (upper left) next to normal liver (bottom right) in a twenty-seven-year-old woman.

RISK FACTORS

Smoking doubles the risk of pancreatic carcinoma (1, 2). Obesity and a high-fat diet have also been associated with an increased risk (1). Pancreatic cancers arise with greater frequency in patients suffering from chronic pancreatitis and diabetes; however, it is sometimes difficult to tell which disease came first, since pancreatic cancer may cause both chronic pancreatitis and diabetes (1, 2).

PERSONAL OBSERVATIONS

My first personal encounter with cancer occurred when my uncle developed pancreatic cancer while I was in high school. He was transformed from a strapping 200-pound man to a 90-pound, skin-covered skeleton in a matter of months. It is a terrible disease! Fortunately, you can minimize your risk with sensible lifestyle choices such as tobacco avoidance, weight maintenance, and a healthy, low-fat diet.

REFERENCES:

1. American Cancer Society. "Cancer Facts & Figures 2007." Atlanta, GA: American Cancer Society, 2007.

2. Hruban RH, Wilentz RE. "The Pancreas." In *Robbins and Cotran Pathologic Basis of Disease*, 7th ed., edited by Kumar et al, 939–53. Philadelphia, PA: Elsevier Saunders, 2005.

2.6: BLADDER CANCER

Each year in the United States about 67,000 cases of bladder cancer are diagnosed, and over 13,000 Americans die of the disease (1). Symptoms of bladder cancer include painful urination, blood in the urine, and increased frequency of urination.

BACKGROUND INFORMATION
The bladder acts as a reservoir for urine produced by the kidneys until urination occurs (Fig. 2.6-1).

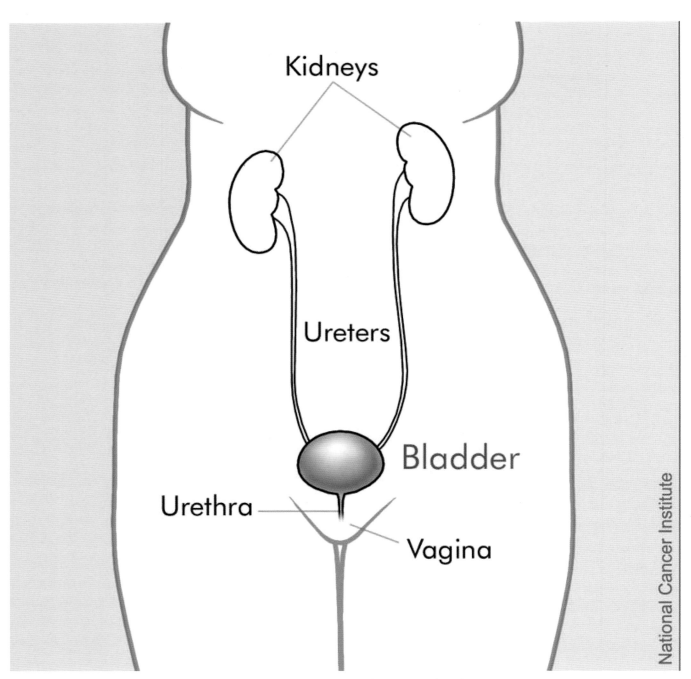

Figure 2.6-1: Location of urinary bladder.
Image courtesy of NIH Medical Arts and National Cancer Institute.

The bladder is lined by a type of epithelium called urothelium (Fig. 2.6-2).

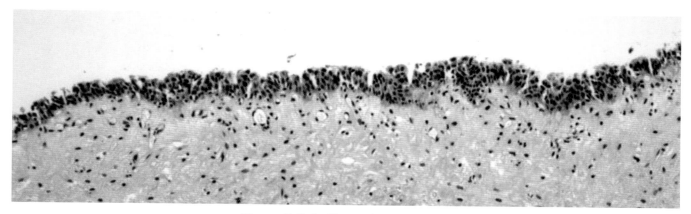

Figure 2.6-2: Normal urothelium.

The underlying bladder wall is composed of loose connective tissue and a muscular wall.

PATHOLOGY

Over 90 percent of bladder cancers arise from the urothelium. The prognosis of these tumors is excellent if invasion of the underlying bladder wall has not occurred. The major types of urothelial carcinoma are low-grade papillary urothelial carcinoma (Fig. 2.6-3), high-grade papillary urothelial carcinoma (Figs. 2.6-4, 2.6-5), and urothelial carcinoma in situ (Fig. 2.6-6).

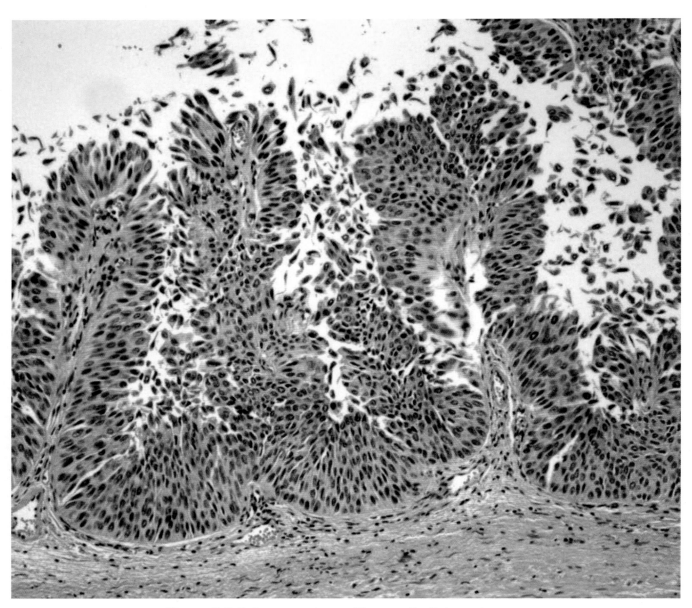

Figure 2.6-3: Low-grade papillary urothelial carcinoma.

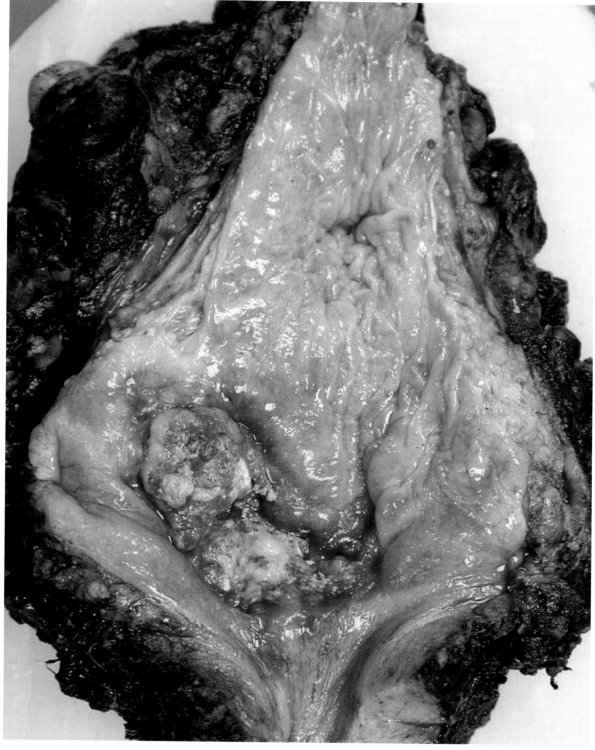

Figure 2.6-4: Opened bladder with high-grade urothelial carcinoma (lower left).

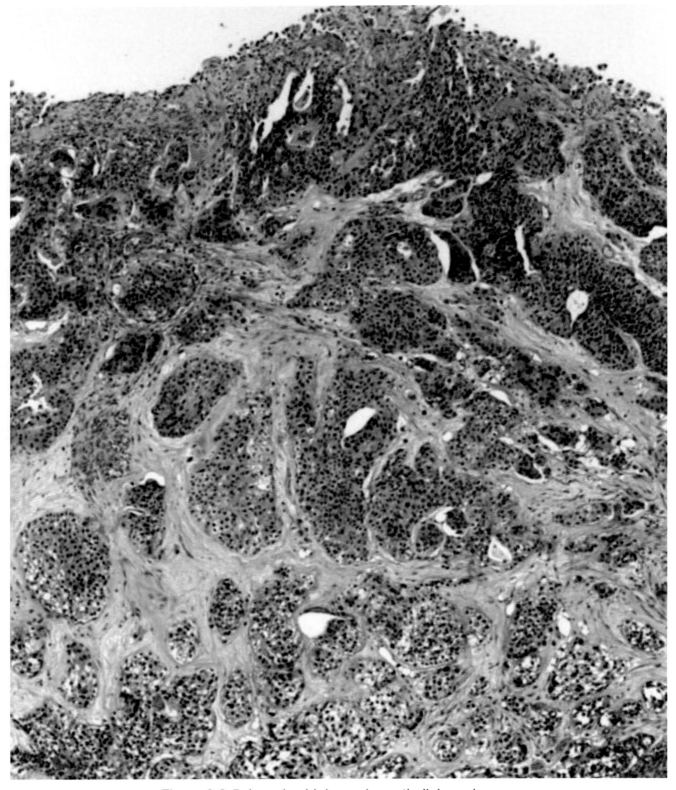

Figure 2.6-5: Invasive high-grade urothelial carcinoma.

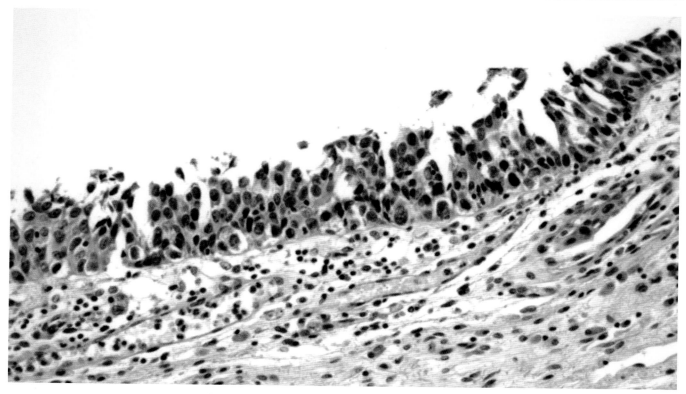

Figure 2.6-6: Urothelial carcinoma in situ.

Invasion of the bladder wall is rare in low-grade papillary urothelial carcinomas, but common in high-grade papillary urothelial carcinomas and urothelial carcinomas in situ. Once invasion of the muscle wall occurs, the five-year survival rate drops to 50 percent (2). In patients with distant metastases, the five-year survival rate drops to 6 percent (1).

Squamous cell carcinoma is a bladder tumor associated with chronic bladder irritation, which makes up between 3 to 7 percent of bladder cancers in the US, but is much more common in countries such as Egypt and Sudan where a parasitic infection called schistosomiasis is common (2). Squamous cell carcinoma of the bladder is an aggressive disease, killing 70 percent of patients within one year (2).

RISK FACTORS

Cigarette smoking is the most prominent risk factor for urothelial carcinomas in the United States, causing 48 percent of bladder cancer deaths in men and 28 percent among women (1). Heavy smokers have up to a sevenfold increased risk over nonsmokers (2). Exposure to industrial chemicals such as 2-Naphthylamine, a chemical used in dye and rubber industries, is also associated with an increased risk (2).

Long-standing chronic inflammation of the bladder, as is seen in patients with chronic indwelling bladder catheters, is also associated with a higher risk of bladder cancer. Most of these cancers are squamous cell carcinomas (2). High vegetable intake may lower the risk of bladder cancer (1).

PERSONAL OBSERVATIONS

When I worked at the University of Missouri, we read biopsies from an adjacent Veterans hospital. Because smoking is very common in military veterans, we saw many cases of bladder cancer. Bladder cancer is yet another reason to avoid smoking. Fortunately, bladder cancer that has not yet invaded the bladder wall can usually be easily and effectively treated. Seek medical attention if you note changes in urination, such as increased frequency, pain, or the presence of blood. While these changes can also be caused by several benign conditions, seeking medical attention at the first sign of these symptoms may allow your doctor an opportunity to detect bladder cancer in an early, curable stage.

REFERENCES:

1. American Cancer Society. "Cancer Facts & Figures 2007." Atlanta, GA: American Cancer Society, 2007.

2. Epstein JI. "The Lower Urinary Tract and Male Genital System." In *Robbins and Cotran Pathologic Basis of Disease*, 7th ed., edited by Kumar et al, 1028–33. Philadelphia, PA: Elsevier Saunders, 2005.

2.7: HEAD AND NECK CANCER

This section will cover the most common malignant tumors of the head and neck, which are carcinomas of the oral cavity (mouth) and larynx (voice box). Approximately 40,000 US cases and more than 500,000 cases worldwide are diagnosed each year (1). Many cases of head and neck cancer present with advanced disease, and the overall long-term survival rate is less than 50 percent (1).

BACKGROUND INFORMATION

The oral cavity and vocal cords are lined by squamous epithelium. Aside from the vocal cords, the healthy larynx is lined by respiratory epithelium. In the presence of chronic irritation (such as the irritation caused by cigarette smoke), the respiratory epithelium will convert into squamous epithelium.

RISK FACTORS AND PATHOLOGY

The main risk factors for head and neck cancer are cigarettes, chewing tobacco, and alcohol ingestion (1, 2). Human papillomavirus (HPV) may also be involved in the development of many of these tumors (1). In India and other parts of Asia, a major predisposing factor is the chewing of betel quid, which is betel leaves filled with various ingredients including areca nut, lime, and tobacco (1). Chronic periodontitis, a gum disease associated with poor dental care, also increases the risk of oral cancers (3). The reason that these risk factors lead to cancers is that they cause damage to the DNA of the squamous cells lining the mouth, throat, and larynx, which in turn can lead to the abnormal growth of these squamous cells. Fortunately, the abnormal growth usually goes through benign phases called hyperkeratosis and dysplasia, which can last for years before a squamous cell carcinoma develops (Figs. 2.7-1 to 2.7-3).

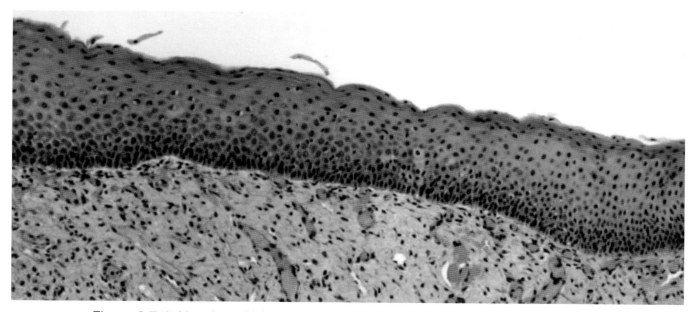

Figure 2.7-1: Vocal cord biopsy showing mild hyperkeratosis but no dysplasia.

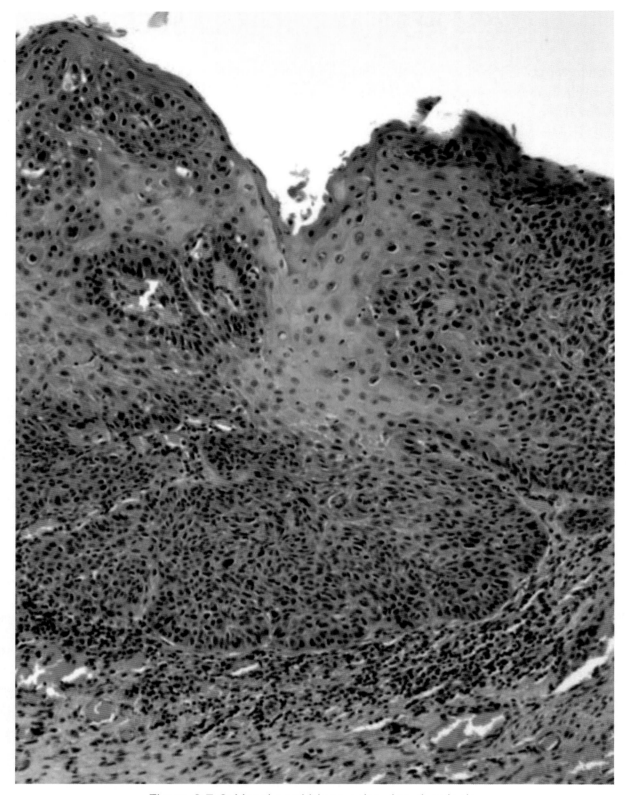

Figure 2.7-2: Vocal cord biopsy showing dysplasia.

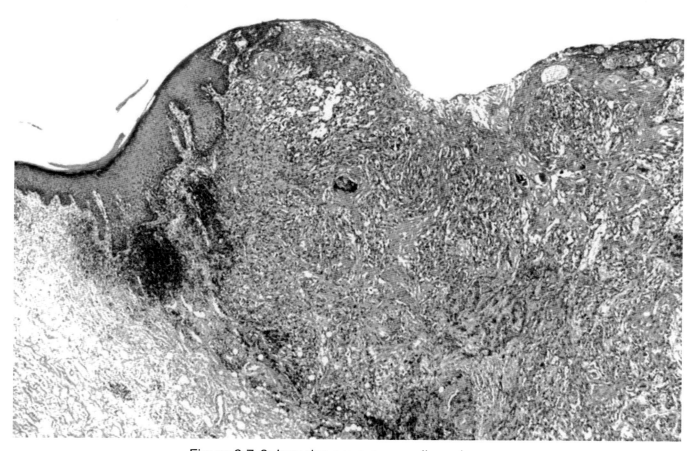

Figure 2.7-3: Invasive squamous cell carcinoma.

These precancerous changes may present as persistent white or red patches in the mouth (Fig. 2.7-4).

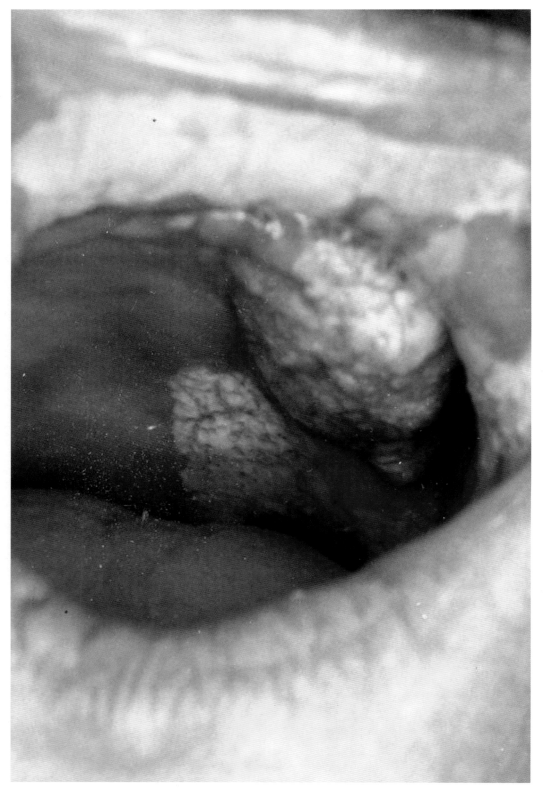

Figure 2.7-4: Squamous cell carcinoma on the roof of the mouth. The white patch toward the back of the mouth represents precancerous dysplasia, while the mass towards the front is invasive carcinoma. Photo courtesy of Steve Westgate, MD.

Similar precancerous changes in the larynx are associated with hoarseness. If the process is caught in this early precancerous stage, it can easily be cured with minimal surgery. Once squamous cell carcinoma develops, the patient may develop large ulcerated masses (Figs. 2.7-5 to 2.7-7).

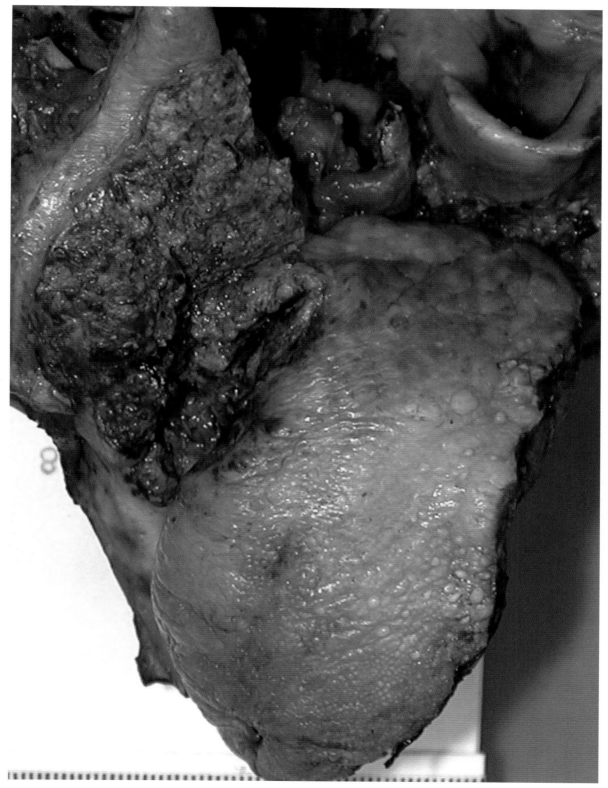

Figure 2.7-5: Surgical resection specimen for squamous cell carcinoma arising next to the tongue.

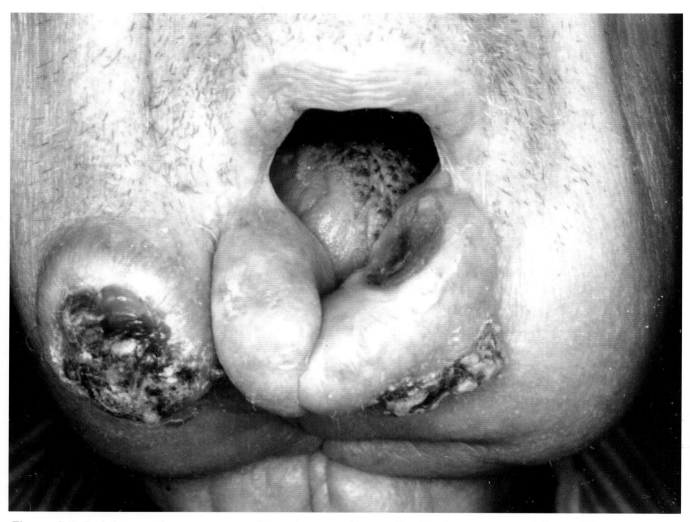

Figure 2.7-6: Advanced squamous cell carcinoma of lower lip. Photo courtesy of Steve Westgate, MD.

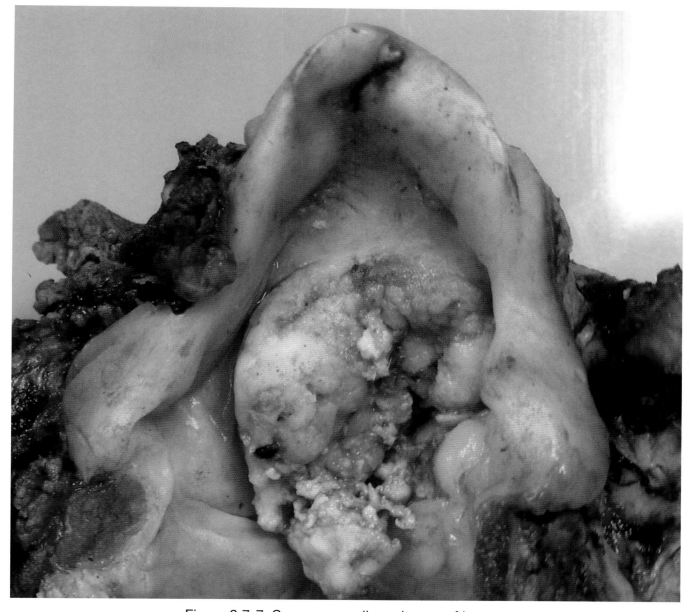

Figure 2.7-7: Squamous cell carcinoma of larynx.

TREATMENT

Surgery and radiation therapy are standard treatments for head and neck cancer. Early detection is important. The surgical removal of precancerous abnormal growths such as hyperkeratosis and dysplasia results in a 100 percent cure rate. About 80 percent of early-stage head and neck cancers can be cured, while only about 19 percent of patients with advanced disease survive.

PERSONAL OBSERVATIONS

Head and neck cancers are often an unwelcome complication when people turn to tobacco and alcohol in order to deal with stress. I've seen many cases where these tumors caused life to go from bad to worse. While head and neck cancers cause significant suffering and death, most can be avoided. If you avoid tobacco and alcohol, your risk of this terrible disease will be greatly reduced. You may also be able to stop this cancer before it fully develops by seeking medical attention for persistent hoarseness or white or red patches in your mouth.

REFERENCES:

1. Lingen MW, Kumar V. "Head and Neck." In *Robbins and Cotran Pathologic Basis of Disease*, 7th ed., edited by Kumar et al, 778–87. Philadelphia, PA: Elsevier Saunders, 2005.

2. American Cancer Society. "Cancer Facts & Figures 2007." Atlanta, GA: American Cancer Society, 2007.

3. Tezal et al. "Chronic Periodontitis and the Incidence of Head and Neck Squamous Cell Carcinoma." *Cancer Epidemiology, Biomarkers & Prevention* 18, no. 9 (2009): 2406–12.

2.8: STOMACH CANCER

Stomach, or gastric, carcinoma is the second-most-common type of cancer worldwide (1). The incidence is especially high in South America, Japan, and China, and is much less common in the United States. Developed countries in general have seen a steady decline of this disease over the past several decades. In 1930, gastric cancer was the most common cause of cancer death in the United States. Over the next seventy years, the mortality rate of the disease in the US dropped from thirty-eight per 100,000 to five per 100,000 (1).

BACKGROUND INFORMATION

Our stomach is an amazing organ. It produces strong acid and enzymes to help digest our food, and has an elaborate system of defense mechanisms that keeps the acid and enzymes from damaging the stomach lining. Three main types of cells are found in the lining of the stomach (Fig. 2.8-1).

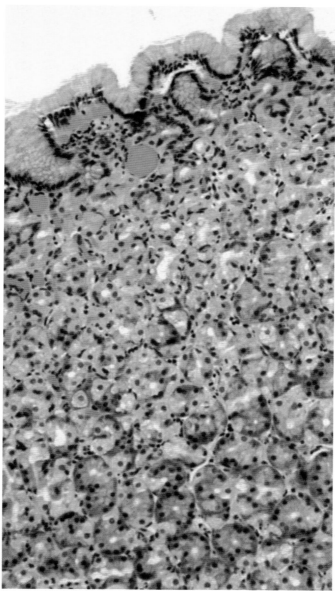

Figure 2.8-1: Normal stomach mucosa. Most cancers arise from the mucus-producing cells lining the lumen (top). Underlying glands include parietal cells (pink) and chief cells (blue).

On the surface, mucus cells secrete mucus, which helps protect our stomach from the acid and digestive enzymes. Parietal cells form gastric acid as well as intrinsic factor, a substance that permits the absorption of vitamin B12. Chief cells make digestive enzymes.

PATHOLOGY

Over 90 percent of gastric cancers are adenocarcinomas, which arise from the mucus cells on the surface of the gastric lining. Gastric adenocarcinomas can show three patterns of growth. Some form an ulcer. Some form a mass that protrudes into the stomach (Fig. 2.8-2).

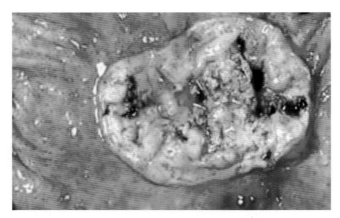

Figure 2.8-2: Adenocarcinoma of stomach, presenting as an ulcerated mass.
Photo courtesy of Alberto Diaz-Arias, MD.

Others cause diffuse thickening of the stomach wall, which is known as linitis plastica (Fig. 2.8-3).

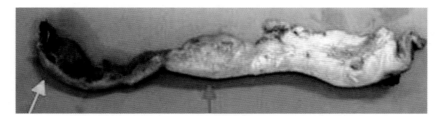

Figure 2.8-3: Cross section of stomach showing the diffuse (linitis plastica) type of adenocarcinoma (pink arrow) adjacent to normal stomach (yellow arrow). Photo courtesy of Alberto Diaz-Arias, MD.

The mass-forming tumors are usually composed of well-developed malignant glands similar to those seen in colon cancer. The diffuse or linitis plastica type of tumors are often made up of sheets of cells resembling a signet ring, which is why they are known as signet-ring cell carcinomas (Figs. 2.8-4, 2.8-5).

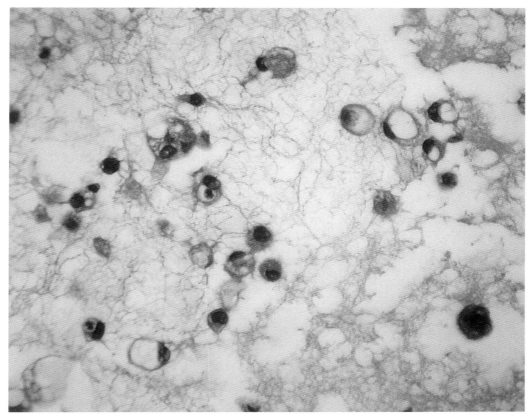

Figure 2.8-4: Signet-ring adenocarcinoma. Photo courtesy of Yale Rosen, MD.

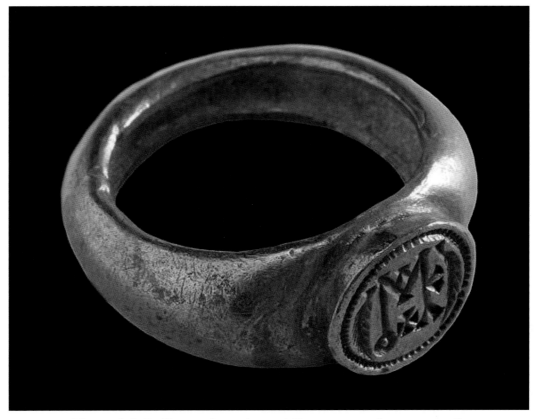

Figure 2.8-5: Signet ring, shaped like a stomach cancer cell.
Public domain image courtesy of Walters Art Museum.

As with most types of carcinomas, the prognosis is closely related to the stage of the disease. Tumors discovered at an early stage with only minimal invasion of the stomach wall show a five-year survival rate of over 90 percent. With advanced gastric cancer, the five-year survival rate drops below 15 percent (1).

RISK FACTORS

Diet: Diet is a major risk factor for stomach cancer and is thought to account for the marked geographic differences in the incidence of this disease. High-risk populations tend to lack refrigeration and have a high intake of preserved, smoked, cured, or salted foods (1). Carcinogens in such foods could play a major role in causing gastric carcinomas. Conversely, diets that include green leafy vegetables and citrus fruits are associated with a decreased risk of gastric carcinoma (1).

Chronic gastritis: Chronic inflammation of the stomach (gastritis) is associated with an increased risk of gastric carcinoma. The most common source of the inflammation is infection with a bacterium known as Helicobacter pylori (Fig. 2.8-6).

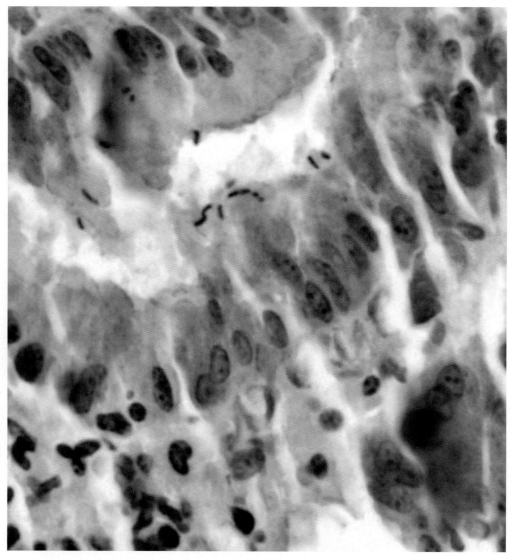

Figure 2.8-6: Helicobacter pylori (wormlike bacteria in center) in a gastric gland.

Helicobacter infections can be treated with antibiotics or Pepto-Bismol. Other common causes of chronic gastritis include the ingestion of toxins such as alcohol and cigarette smoke, and autoimmune gastritis, a disease where the body's immune system attacks the parietal cells (1).

Regardless of the cause, chronic gastritis is frequently associated with symptoms such as belching, feeling full or bloated, nausea, vomiting, and dark, sticky stools. The mucosa in chronic gastritis often goes through a sequence of benign changes including atrophy, intestinal metaplasia, and dysplasia before carcinoma develops. While benign, dysplasia is a precancerous growth of the gastric lining cells. Surgical excision of the gastric dysplasia can prevent stomach cancers before they form.

PERSONAL OBSERVATIONS

The vast majority of cases of gastric adenocarcinoma that I have seen have been associated with very sad stories. Most cases have advanced disease and a very poor prognosis by the time they come to medical attention. Fortunately, the risk of this disease can be greatly reduced with general healthy lifestyle choices. Seek medical attention if you have symptoms associated with gastritis. Most cases of gastritis are caused by Helicobacter infections, which can be easily treated. Eat a healthy diet with abundant fruits and vegetables. Avoid smoked, cured, or salted meat products.

REFERENCE:

1. Liu C, Crawford JM. "The Gastrointestinal Tract." In *Robbins and Cotran Pathologic Basis of Disease*, 7th ed., edited by Kumar et al, 812–26. Philadelphia, PA: Elsevier Saunders, 2005.

2.9: ENDOMETRIAL CANCER

Each year about 39,000 US women are diagnosed with endometrial cancer and over 7,000 US women die of the disease (1). Endometrial carcinoma (Figs. 2.9-1 to 2.9-3) is currently the most common invasive cancer of the female genital tract (2).

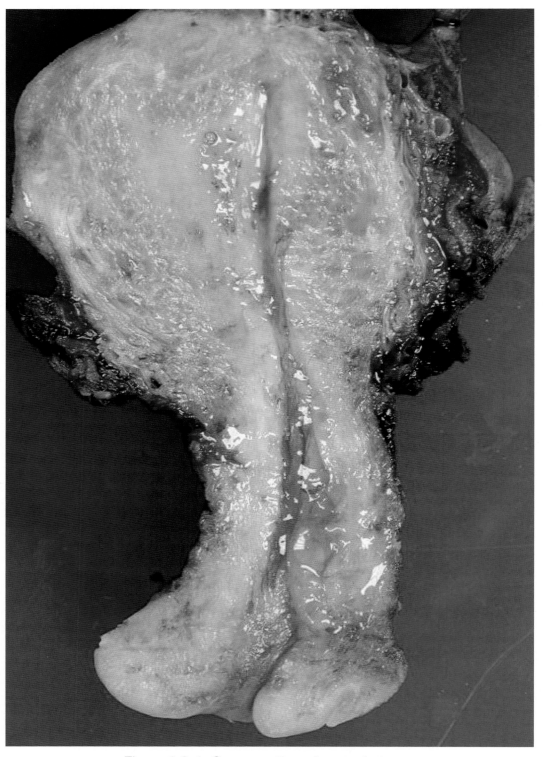

Figure 2.9-1: Cross section of normal uterus.

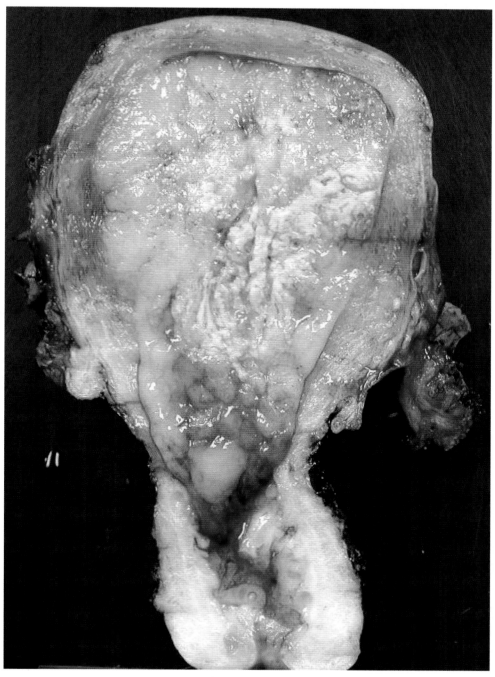

Figure 2.9-2: Cross section of uterus with endometrial adenocarcinoma.

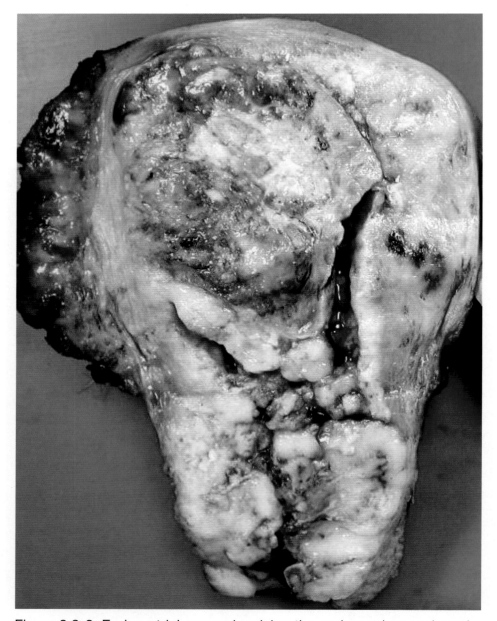

Figure 2.9-3: Endometrial cancer involving the endometrium and cervix.

Endometrial carcinoma is uncommon in women younger than forty years old, and is often discovered in women who experience postmenopausal bleeding.

BACKGROUND INFORMATION

The endometrium is the lining of the uterus, and supports the implantation of embryos. The lining is normally shed during a woman's monthly menstrual cycle. The first half of the cycle is called the proliferative phase, and is associated with rapid growth of endometrial tissue under the influence of estrogen. After ovulation, a structure called a corpus luteum, which produces progesterone, develops in the ovaries. Under the influence of progesterone, the endometrium undergoes its secretory phase. If pregnancy does not occur, progesterone levels drop and sloughing of the endometrium occurs— otherwise known as menstruation. The female hormone cycle is closely regulated by the body; most premenopausal women have fairly regular cycles that last approximately twenty-eight days.

PATHOLOGY

Most endometrial cancers are adenocarcinomas, which resemble proliferative endometrium (endometrioid adenocarcinoma) (Figs. 2.9-4 to 2.9-6). In most cases, endometrial carcinomas arise in benign but precancerous endometrial proliferations called endometrial hyperplasia.

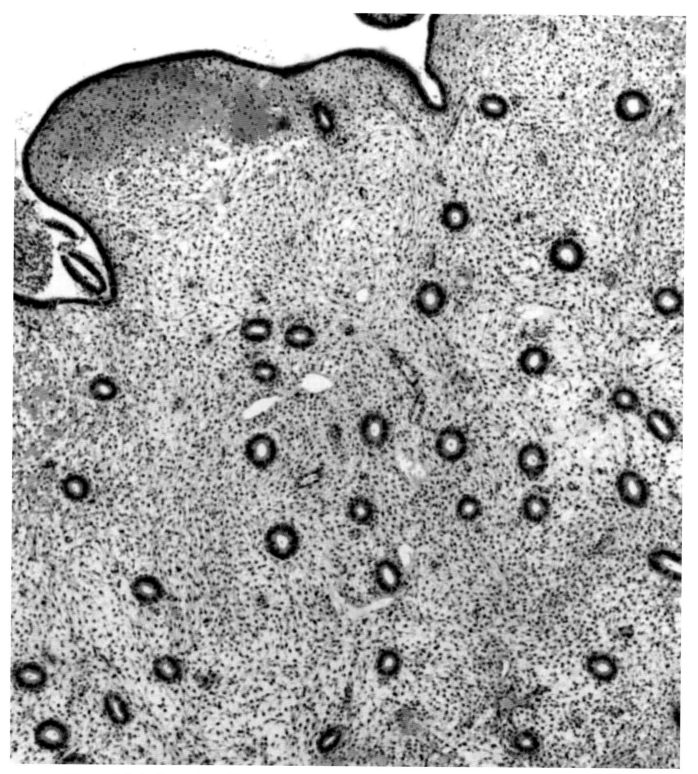

Figure 2.9-4: Normal proliferative endometrium with uniformly spaced tubular glands.

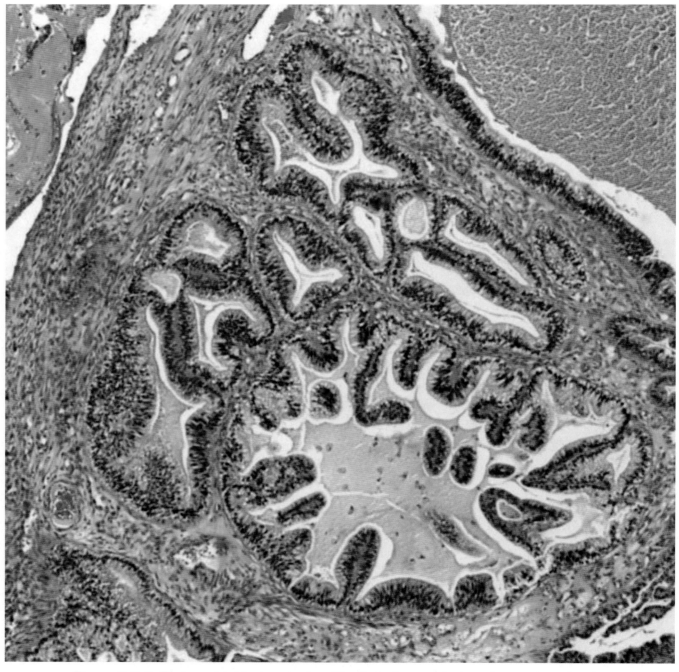

Figure 2.9-5: Endometrial hyperplasia with dilated, crowded, and complex glands.

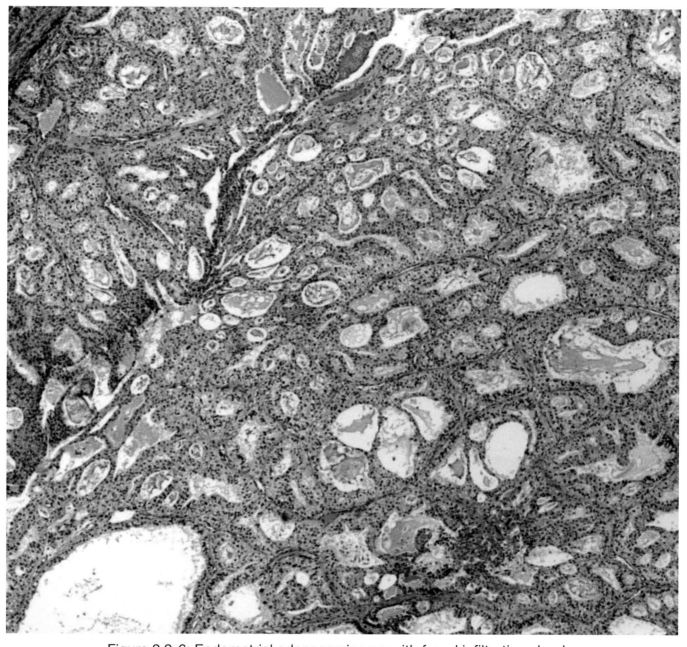

Figure 2.9-6: Endometrial adenocarcinoma with fused infiltrative glands.

Abnormal uterine bleeding, especially postmenopausal bleeding, is a sign of both endometrial hyperplasia and carcinoma.

Endometrial hyperplasia can be cured with hormonal therapy or surgery. As with the other carcinomas, the survival rate of endometrial carcinoma is closely related to the stage of the disease. The five-year survival rate for typical endometrioid adenocarcinoma is 96 percent if caught at an early stage. If distant metastases have occurred, the five-year survival rate drops to 23 percent (1).

RISK FACTORS

Unopposed estrogen stimulation (estrogen without progesterone) is the major risk factor for endometrioid adenocarcinoma (1). Estrogen stimulates the endometrium to grow, while progesterone inhibits endometrial proliferation. As a result, women on hormone-replacement therapy who only take estrogen increase their risk of endometrioid adenocarcinoma. Conversely, using combined estrogen/progesterone therapy does not significantly increase the risk (1).

Obesity is also associated with an increased risk of endometrial cancer. The increased risk of endometrial cancer seen in obesity is due to the increased estrogen levels that occur from the conversion of adrenal hormones to estrogen in body fat.

Pregnancy and the use of oral contraceptives have been associated with a decreased risk of this type of cancer (1).

PERSONAL OBSERVATIONS

Many women do not like to go to the doctor and discuss abnormal menstrual bleeding. While this is understandable, it can also lead to dangerous behavior. Failure to seek medical attention for abnormal bleeding was a major factor in the presentation of most of the advanced endometrial cancers I saw in my pathology practice. Endometrial cancer is another example of a serious disease that can often be avoided through lifestyle changes and proper medical treatment. You can significantly decrease your risk if you avoid unopposed estrogen therapy and obesity. Seek prompt medical attention for abnormal menstrual bleeding, especially postmenopausal bleeding. Early medical attention in response to abnormal bleeding can detect endometrial hyperplasia or early noninvasive cancers, which can be easily cured.

REFERENCES:

1. American Cancer Society. "Cancer Facts & Figures 2007." Atlanta, GA: American Cancer Society, 2007.

2. Crum C. "The Female Genital Tract." In *Robbins and Cotran Pathologic Basis of Disease*, 7th ed., edited by Kumar et al, 1059–89. Philadelphia, PA: Elsevier Saunders, 2005.

2.10: SKIN CANCER

The skin is the most common site of cancer in Caucasians. The two most common types of skin cancers are basal cell carcinoma and squamous cell carcinoma. These tumors can usually be cured by simple excision. Melanoma, the third-most-common type of skin cancer, is a more aggressive tumor, which is much more likely to metastasize to other areas of the body. Each year, over 1 million new cases of skin cancer, including approximately 60,000 cases of melanoma, are diagnosed in the United States (1). Each year, over 10,000 Americans die from skin cancer, and over 8,000 of these deaths are due to melanoma (1).

BACKGROUND INFORMATION

The skin is made up of an outer layer of epidermis with underlying dermis. The epidermis is composed mainly of squamous cells. At the base of the epidermis are scattered melanocytes (Figs. 2.10-1A, 2.10-1B).

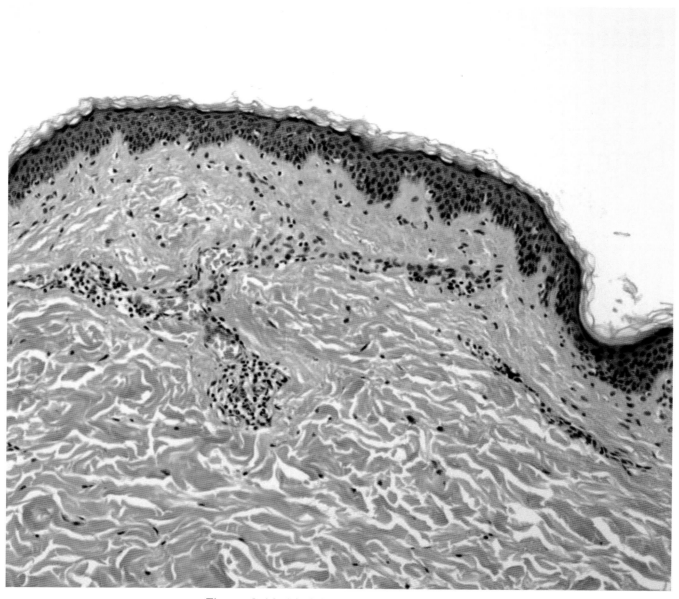

Figure 2.10-1A: Histology of normal skin.

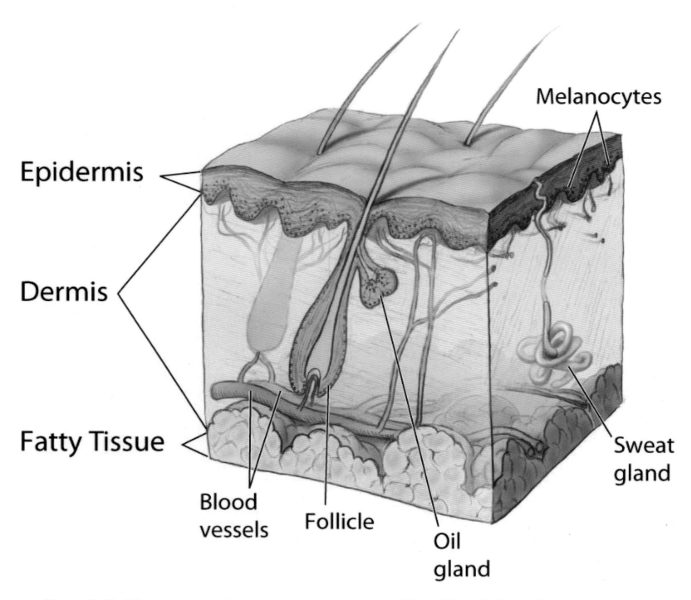

Figure 2.10-1B: Anatomy of the skin. Image courtesy of Don Bliss, National Cancer Institute.

Melanocytes are cells that produce melanin pigment, which acts as a screen against the harmful ultraviolet (UV) rays that come from sunlight. Also present in the epidermis are Langerhans cells. Langerhans cells help the immune system recognize and fight infections or cancer cells.

PATHOLOGY

Basal cell carcinomas (Fig. 2.10-2) and squamous cell carcinomas (Fig. 2.10-3) are the two most common types of skin cancer.

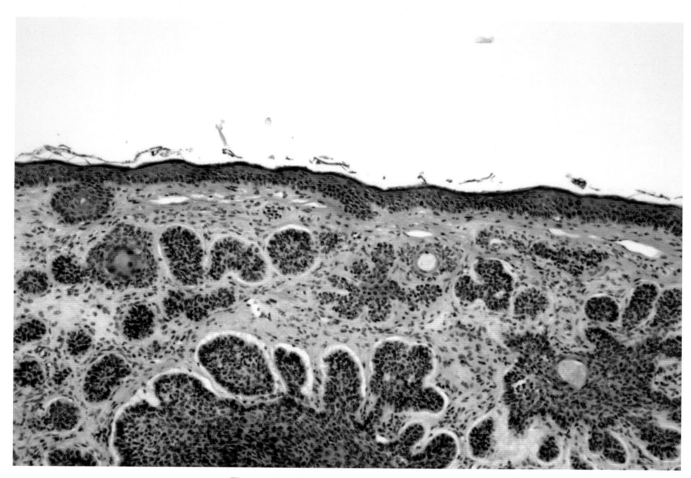

Figure 2.10-2: Basal cell carcinoma.

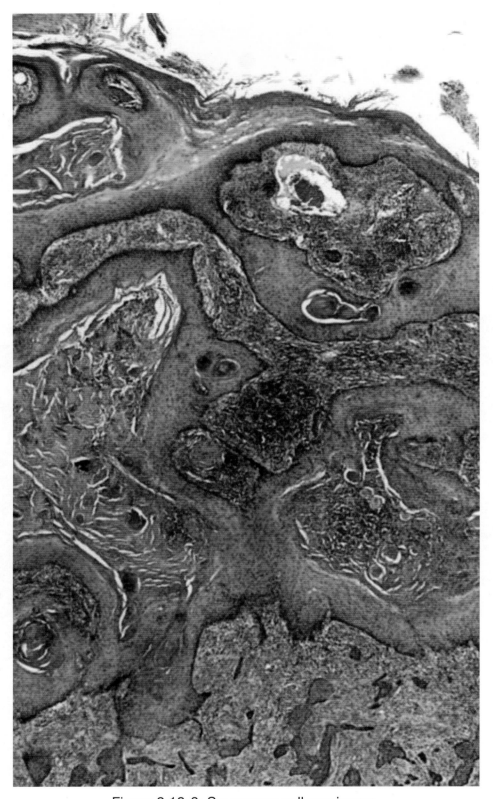

Figure 2.10-3: Squamous cell carcinoma.

Both types arise from the squamous cells in the epidermis. These tumors, particularly squamous cell carcinomas, sometimes develop in a benign precursor lesion called actinic keratosis. Detected early, cutaneous basal cell carcinoma and squamous cell carcinoma are readily cured by local excision. If neglected, these tumors can be locally aggressive and even metastasize (Figs. 2.10-4 to 2.10-6).

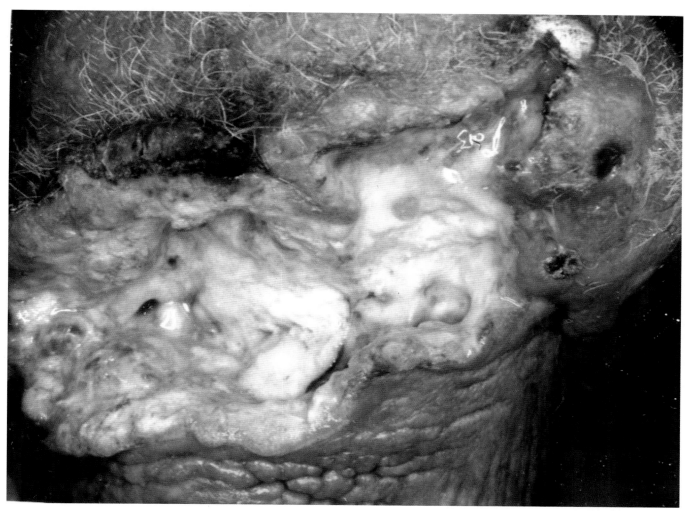

Figure 2.10-4: Advanced skin cancer on back of neck. Photo courtesy of Steve Westgate, MD.

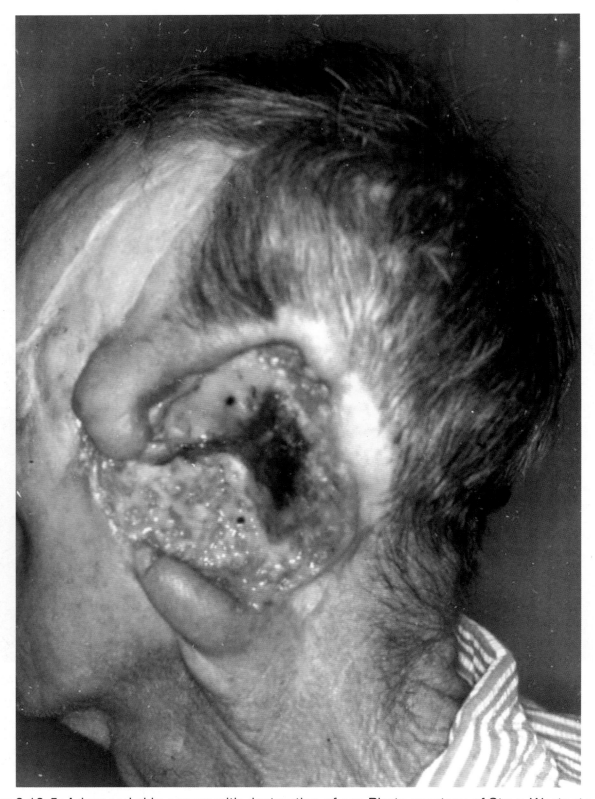

Figure 2.10-5: Advanced skin cancer with destruction of ear. Photo courtesy of Steve Westgate, MD.

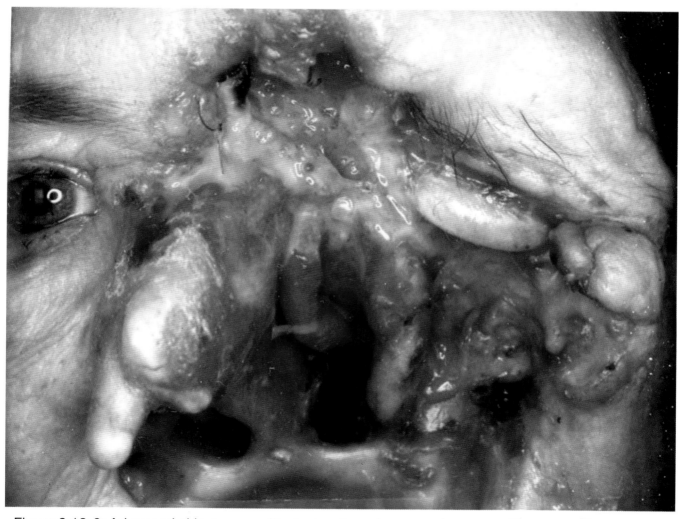

Figure 2.10-6: Advanced skin cancer with destruction of nose and one eye. Photo courtesy of Steve Westgate, MD.

Melanomas arise from the melanocytes present at the base of the epidermis. They usually have an initial phase of noninvasive growth called melanoma in situ, which is readily cured by local excision (Fig. 2.10-7).

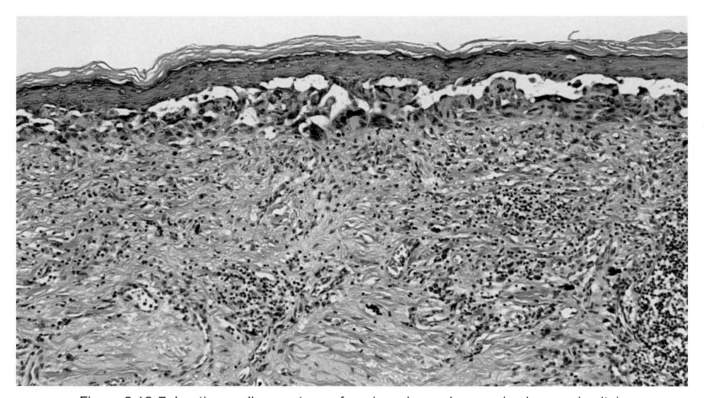

Figure 2.10-7: Lentigo maligna, a type of noninvasive melanoma (melanoma in situ).

The prognosis of melanoma declines rapidly with the increasing depth of invasion into the dermis. While over 90 percent of tumors with a depth of invasion less than 1 millimeter will be cured by excision, most people with ulcerated tumors invading deeper than 4 millimeters will die of metastatic disease. Invasion can be rapid once it occurs. Although most melanomas invade about 0.12 millimeters per month, one-third invade 0.5 or more millimeters per month (3). This data underscores the importance of early detection and treatment. Delay of a few months can literally make the difference between life and death.

Basal cell carcinomas may appear as flat, firm, pale areas or as small, raised, shiny areas with prominent blood vessels (1) (Fig. 2.10-8).

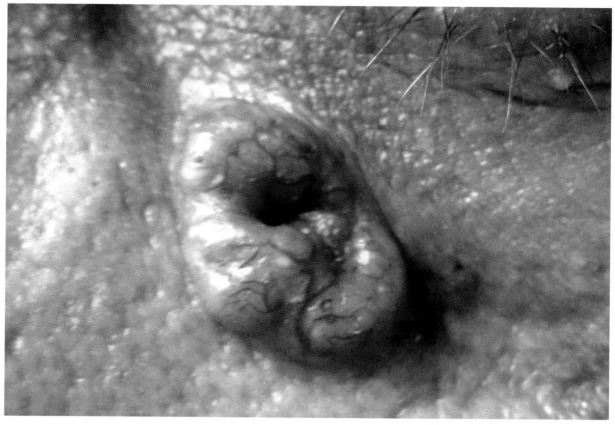

Figure 2.10-8: Basal cell carcinoma. Photo courtesy of Michelle Wanna, MD.

Squamous cell carcinomas may look like flat, reddish patches or nodular lumps with a rough, ulcerated surface (1) (Fig. 2.10-9).

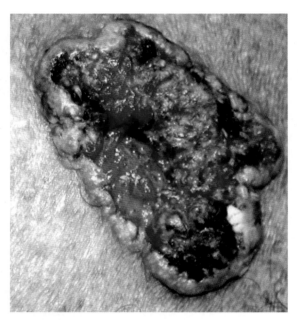

Figure 2.10-9: Squamous cell carcinoma. Photo courtesy of Mary Feldman, MD.

Warning signs for melanoma are outlined by a simple ABCD rule (1) (Fig. 2.10-10 to 2.10-12):

A. Asymmetry (one half of the mole does not match the other half)
B. Border irregularity
C. Color pigmentation is not a uniform brown or includes areas of red, white, or blue
D. Diameter greater than 6 millimeters

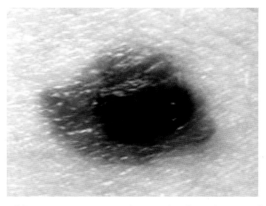

Figure 2.10-10: Early melanoma. Note asymmetry, irregular border, and color variation. Photo courtesy of Holly Hare, MD.

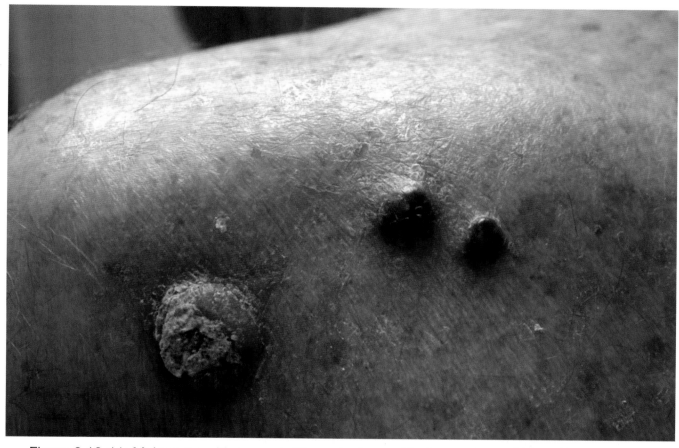

Figure 2.10-11: Melanoma with two satellite metastases. Photo courtesy of Mary Feldman, MD.

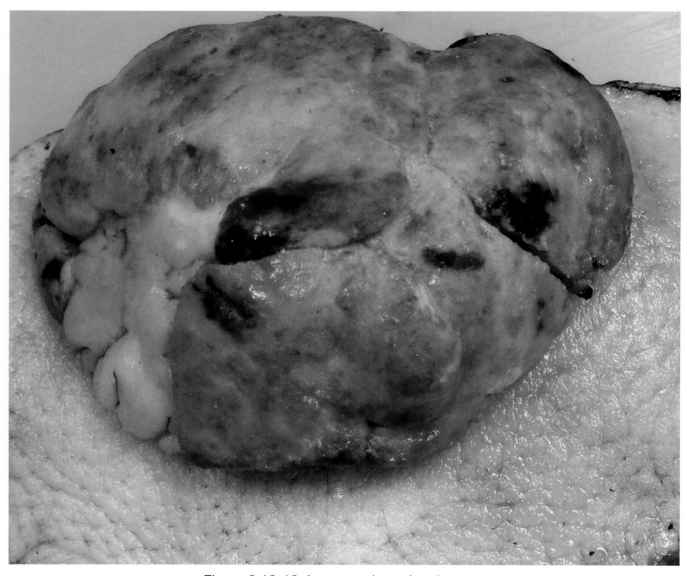

Figure 2.10-12: Large neglected melanoma
(diameter 6.5 cm/thickness 20 mm).

It is important to note that some melanomas don't produce pigment and can simulate other skin lesions (Fig. 2.10-13).

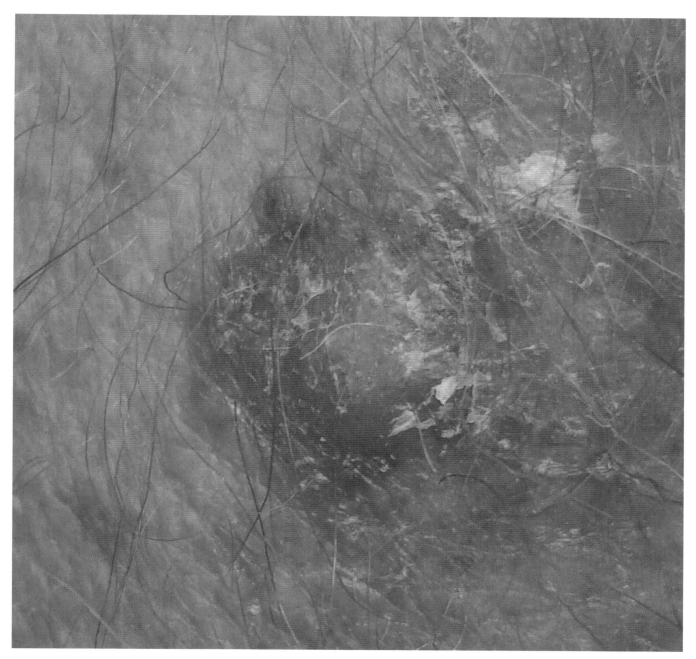

Figure 2.10-13: Amelanotic melanoma. Not all melanomas are pigmented.
Photo courtesy of Holly Hare, MD.

It is very important to seek prompt medical attention for any persistent skin lesion, particularly if it is growing or changing. The best treatment for any skin cancer is surgical excision. The earlier a skin cancer is treated, the simpler the treatment and the better the prognosis. Excision of an early, small skin cancer is nearly painless, and is associated with a nearly 100 percent cure rate. If you delay seeking medical attention, the prognosis is worse, and the treatment can be more complicated and painful.

RISK FACTORS

Sun exposure: Sun exposure is the most frequent cause of skin cancers. Sunlight includes three types of harmful ultraviolet (UV) radiation: UVA, UVB, and UVC. UVC is the most dangerous type of ultraviolet radiation. Fortunately, it is completely filtered by ozone in the atmosphere and doesn't reach earth. (Ever wonder why preserving the ozone layer is important?) While the atmosphere absorbs the UVC rays, most of the UVA rays and about 10 percent of the UVB rays reach the earth's surface. The UV radiation reaching earth consists of 95 percent UVA and 5 percent UVB. UVA rays are responsible for most of the features of aging skin, such as wrinkles, and cause some skin cancers. UVB rays are the main cause of sunburn and cause most skin cancers. Tanning beds work by emitting UVA and UVB radiation. Most tanning beds predominantly emit UVA rays. However, in recent years, some tanning beds have been made to also emit significant levels of UVB to speed the tanning process. Regardless of the source, ultraviolet radiation causes skin cancer by damaging the DNA in skin cells. It has been estimated that exposure to midday sun can produce up to 40,000 DNA errors per hour. While the body has elaborate repair processes to fix most of these DNA errors, chronic exposure to strong ultraviolet radiation can overwhelm the system. In addition to damaging DNA, ultraviolet radiation is also thought to have an immunosuppressive effect on Langerhans cells in the epidermis, which hinders the immune system's response to developing tumors (2). Dark-skinned individuals have more melanin in their skin to help prevent damage from ultraviolet radiation. Thus, melanoma rates are more than ten times higher in Caucasians than in African Americans (1). Fair-skinned individuals who sunburn easily are particularly prone to developing skin cancer. Prolonged exposure to ultraviolet radiation—either from the sunlight, particularly during midday hours, or tanning beds—increases the risk of these tumors.

Occupational exposure to carcinogens: Exposure to cold tar, pitch, creosote, arsenic, or radium is associated with an increased risk of skin cancers (1). While sun exposure is the most important risk factor for skin cancers, I have seen cases where these tumors developed in skin that was chronically exposed to carcinogenic substances. One case was a construction worker who developed a skin cancer on the shoulder that he used to carry lumber treated with arsenic and creosote. Early in my career, I looked at skin biopsies from an elderly veteran who had been exposed to arsenic-containing chemical weapons during World War I and developed numerous basal cell carcinomas many years later.

Family history: Several familial syndromes are associated with an increased risk of skin cancer. Most of these are due to genetic mutations, which promote tumor development. For example, people with a condition called xeroderma pigmentosum have a diminished capacity to repair DNA after exposure to ultraviolet radiation. This leads to a high incidence of skin cancers, which often develop in young children.

Immunosuppression: Patients with suppressed immune systems due to genetic defects, those with infections such as HIV, or those who are on certain kinds of medication (such as the type commonly prescribed to transplant patients) have an increased risk of developing skin cancer. One study found that 48 percent of patients undergoing kidney transplantation later developed skin cancer.

PREVENTION

The most effective way to prevent skin cancer is to minimize your exposure to ultraviolet (UV) radiation found in sunlight and tanning beds. Practical ways to do this, according to the World Health Organization, include:

1. Limit time in the midday sun. The sun's UV rays are strongest between 10 a.m. and 4 p.m.
2. Seek shade. While trees, umbrellas, etc., do not completely protect you from UV radiation, they certainly help. If you are in bright enough sun to cast a shadow, look for more shade.
3. Wear protective clothing. Hats with wide brims can provide good protection for your head and neck. Loose-fitting clothing can be a comfortable way to protect the rest of your body. Sunglasses can help protect your eyes from UV-induced diseases such as cataracts. According to the American National Standards Institute, sunglasses must block over 60 percent of UVA radiation and 95 percent of UVB.
4. Avoid sunlamps and tanning beds.
5. Use sunscreen on exposed skin. Sunscreens are typically rated with a sun protection factor (SPF). SPF numbers are based on the following equation: Minutes to burn without sunscreen x SPF # = maximum exposure time without burn

For example, if you would naturally burn after twenty minutes of sun exposure, an SPF 10 sunscreen would allow you to be in the sun for 200 minutes before burning. SPF numbers provide a measure of protection from UVB radiation (Table 2.10A), but do not relate to UVA protection. Mexoryl SX, also known as ecamsule, is a particularly good UVA-blocking ingredient found in some sunscreens.

TABLE 2.10A
RELATIONSHIP BETWEEN SPF RATING AND UVB ABSORPTION

SPF	% UVB Blocked
2	50
4	70
8	87.5
15	93.3
30	96.7
50	98

It is important to note that a tan provides only limited protection against UV radiation and sunburns. A dark tan in a light-skinned individual is about equivalent to an SPF 3 sunscreen.

PERSONAL OBSERVATIONS

We have a great opportunity to eliminate most of the pain and suffering caused by skin cancers. Your risk of these tumors can be greatly reduced by following the prevention guidelines in this chapter. Early treatment can easily cure those skin cancers that do form in spite of preventive measures. Tumors of the skin can be readily detected by physical examination, and the time of the diagnosis can literally make the difference between life and death. I've seen many advanced cases of melanoma that could have been easily cured if the patient had sought medical attention earlier. While basal cell carcinomas and squamous cell carcinomas are more indolent, they should not be neglected. I've seen cases where they grew through the skull into the brain or invaded the deep tissue of an arm, requiring amputation. Examine your skin regularly for any discolorations or lesions like those described in this chapter. Seek medical help promptly for anything suspicious.

REFERENCES:

1. American Cancer Society. "Cancer Facts & Figures 2007." Atlanta, GA: American Cancer Society, 2007.

2. Murphy et al. "The Skin." In *Robbins and Cotran Pathologic Basis of Disease*, 7th ed., edited by Kumar et al, 1227–47. Philadelphia, PA: Elsevier Saunders, 2005.

3. Liu et al. "Rate of Growth in Melanomas: Characteristics and Associations of Rapidly Growing Melanomas." *Archives of Dermatology* 142 (2006): 1551–58.

3: CHRONIC OBSTRUCTIVE PULMONARY DISEASE

Chronic obstructive pulmonary disease (COPD) is the third-most-common killer in the United States after atherosclerosis and cancer. Over 120,000 US citizens and approximately 2.7 million people worldwide die from this disorder each year (1). The two forms of COPD—emphysema and chronic bronchitis— often appear in the same patient, as both forms are caused primarily by cigarette smoking (2).

BACKGROUND INFORMATION

The lungs are perfectly formed to allow for the necessary exchange of gases between inhaled air and blood. Air enters the lungs through rigid cartilage-lined tubes called bronchi. The bronchi subdivide into more flexible bronchioles, which lack cartilage. The bronchioles further subdivide into tubes of an increasingly smaller diameter until the air comes in contact with tiny air sacs called alveoli (Fig. 3-1).

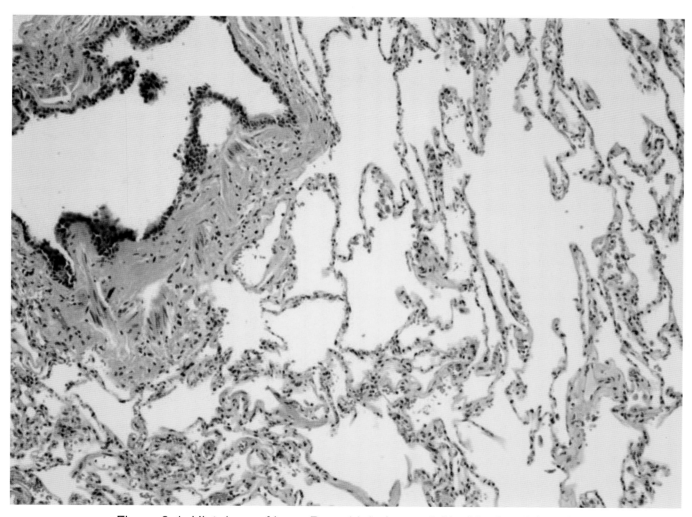

Figure 3-1: Histology of lung: Bronchiole (upper left) with alveoli (right).

Alveoli are lined by a single layer of epithelial cells and have walls formed by thin-walled blood vessels called capillaries (Fig. 3-2).

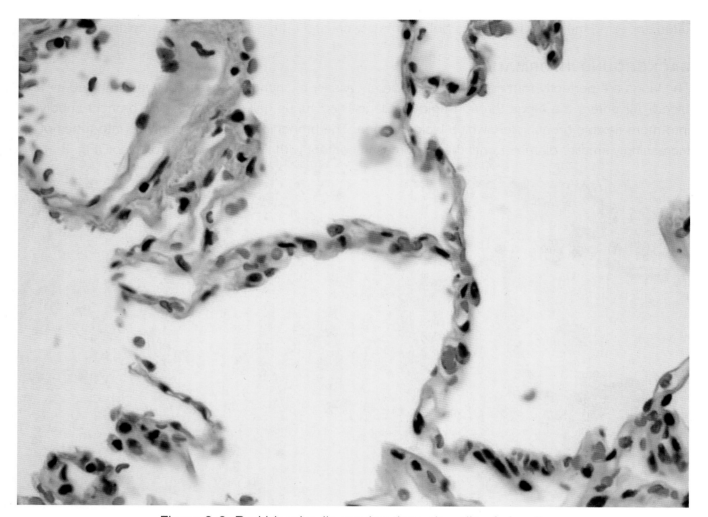

Figure 3-2: Red blood cells moving through walls of alveoli.

The exchange of oxygen and carbon dioxide occurs across this thin alveolar-capillary membrane with each breath.

PATHOLOGY

Emphysema is characterized by abnormally enlarged air spaces due to the destruction of alveolar walls (Fig. 3-3).

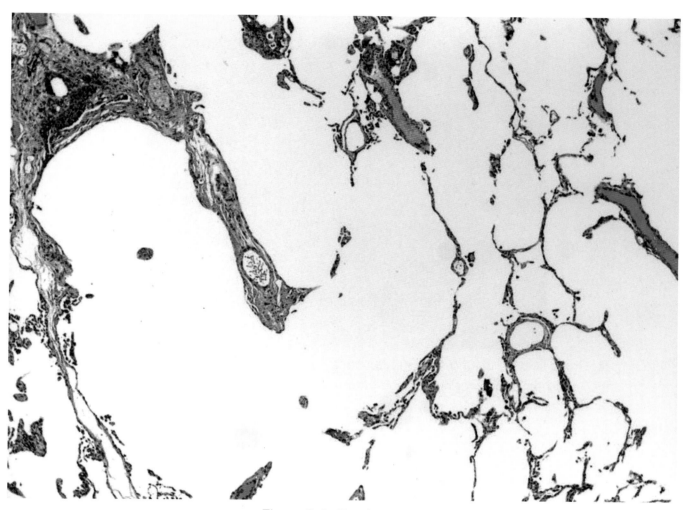

Figure 3-3: Emphysema.

Cigarette smoke stimulates inflammatory cells to release substances normally used to fight infection, such as protease, elastase, and oxygen-free radicals. Tobacco smoke itself also contains numerous oxygen-free radicals. These substances work together to eat away at normal lung tissue. Cigarette smoke also depletes the lung of alpha-1 antitrypsin, a substance that inactivates potentially damaging substances released with inflammation (2).

Air gets trapped in the abnormal dilated air spaces found in emphysema (Fig. 3-4), and the normal exchange of oxygen and carbon dioxide does not occur properly.

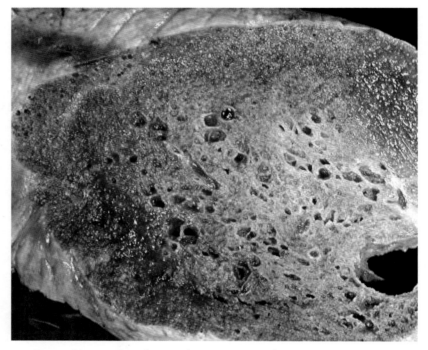

Figure 3-4: Cross section of lung showing pulmonary emphysema. Note enlarged air spaces in the center and lower right of the photo compared to the rest of the lung.

Eventually, large bubble-like air spaces called bulla are formed (Fig. 3-5).

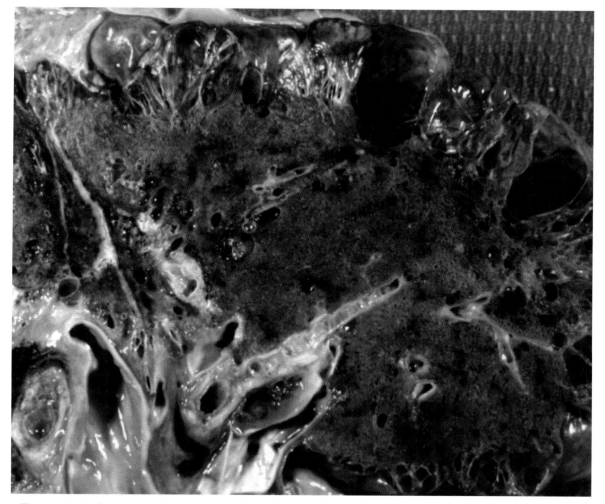

Figure 3-5: Cross section of lung showing emphysema with peripheral bulla (top right).
Photo courtesy of Ann Havey, MD.

Bulla sometimes rupture, causing the lung to deflate like a popped balloon.

In chronic bronchitis, cigarette smoke or other inhaled irritants stimulate increased mucin production of the cells lining the bronchi and bronchioles. The result is mucus plugs, which stop airflow; an infection is usually close behind (2).

Emphysema usually results in a shortness of breath known as dyspnea. Symptoms do not usually appear until over one-third of the lung tissue has been damaged. Chronic bronchitis is characterized by a persistent cough, where the patient coughs up the excess mucin produced in his or her airway. In both conditions, continued exposure to the offending agent often leads to progressive respiratory failure and death.

RISK FACTORS
Smoking causes 90 percent of chronic obstructive pulmonary disease (2). In addition to affecting smokers, emphysema can develop in patients with a genetic deficiency of alpha-1 antitrypsin. In addition to tobacco, chronic bronchitis can result from inhaling irritants such as grain, cotton, and silica dust (2). Lung disease from these dusts are most commonly seen in workers in grain elevators and grain mills,

textile workers, miners, and sandblasters. If you work in a dusty environment, be sure to wear a dust mask or respirator.

PERSONAL OBSERVATIONS

Most smokers fear dying from lung cancer. Many lung specialists say that they should fear COPD more. People with end-stage COPD have chronic shortness of breath that simulates drowning. It is a terrible disease. I've seen many lungs from surgical resections and autopsies that had such extensive damage that I had to wonder how any respiration occurred.

Fortunately, COPD is another example of a common, devastating disease that could be greatly reduced by making lifestyle changes. Avoid smoking and you decrease your risk by 90 percent. Smoking cessation can also prevent the progression of the disease and improve lung function. While emphysema causes permanent destruction of lung tissue, most patients with COPD have a reversible component of chronic bronchitis that will go away when they stop smoking.

REFERENCES:

1. COPD International. Last modified March 16, 2004. www.copd-international.com.

2. Husain AN, Kumar V. "The Lung." In *Robbins and Cotran Pathologic Basis of Disease*, 7th ed., edited by Kumar et al, 717–23. Philadelphia, PA: Elsevier Saunders, 2005.

4: ACCIDENTS

Now, for a slight change of pace. Though not a type of disease, accidents are the fourth leading cause of death in the United States after atherosclerosis, cancer, and chronic obstructive pulmonary disease (1). Over 85,000 Americans die from accidents each year (2). The top five causes of accidental death in the US are motor vehicle accidents (over 43,000 per year), poisoning (over 27,000 per year), falls (nearly 15,000 per year), fires (approximately 3,700 per year), and drowning (approximately 3,500 per year) (2,12). The majority of these are preventable.

MOTOR VEHICLE ACCIDENTS

Worldwide, since cars were invented, more than 25 million people have died in motor vehicle accidents. Currently, about 1.2 million die each year on the roads (3). The tremendous force of these accidents can break structures such as the aorta (Figs. 4-1, 4-2) and the spinal cord (Fig. 4-3) in half.

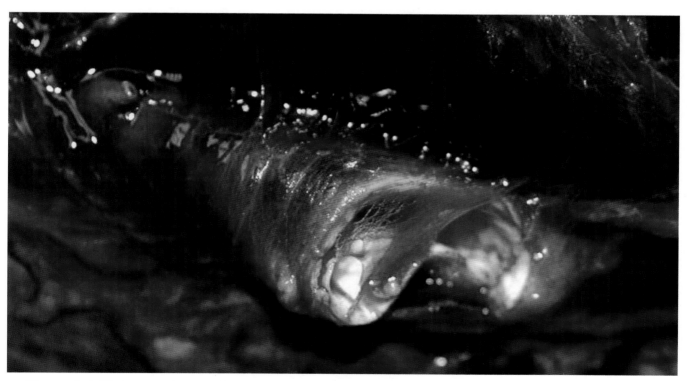

Figure 4-1: Transected aorta due to motor vehicle accident. Photo courtesy of Mike Panella, MD.

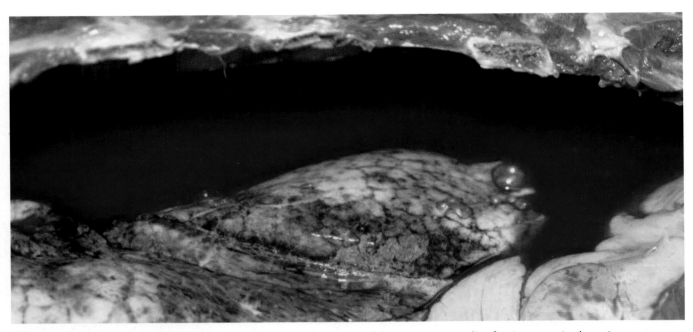

Figure 4-2: Hemorrhage in chest cavity around lung as a result of a transected aorta.
Photo courtesy of Mike Panella, MD.

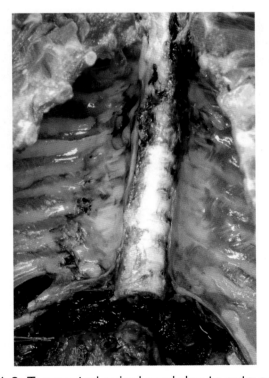

Figure 4-3: Transected spinal cord due to auto accident.

In the United States, motor vehicle–related injury is the leading cause of death for people ages one to thirty-four (4). Each year, about 5 million US citizens experience traffic accidents that require an emergency room visit, at a cost of about $230 billion (Figs. 4-4, 4-5) (4).

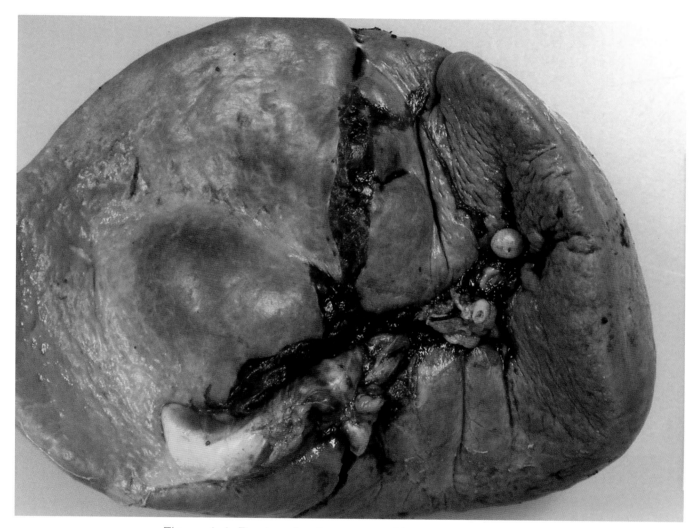

Figure 4-4: Ruptured spleen caused by an auto accident.

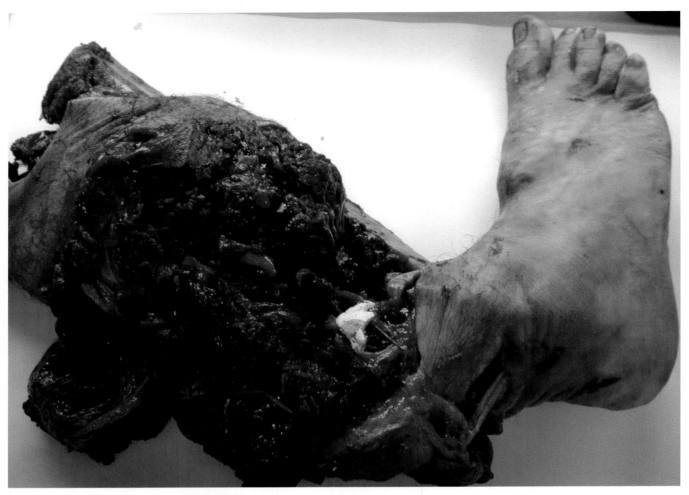

Figure 4-5: Amputation specimen due to motor vehicle accident.

Nearly 80 percent of auto accidents in the US are caused when a driver becomes inattentive due to distracting activities or drowsiness (5). Distracting activities associated with increased risk include using your cell phone; reaching for a moving object, such as paperwork falling off the passenger seat; looking at something that takes your eyes off the road, such as a car accident on the other side of the highway; reading; and applying makeup. Each time you take your eyes off the road is an opportunity to be a statistic. Stay focused on driving!

Drowsiness is estimated to cause at least 100,000 traffic accidents each year in the United States (3). This is not surprising, since nearly 20 percent of the adults in our country report excessive sleepiness, and 17.7 percent report drowsiness or falling asleep in situations requiring high concentration (9). Most of the remaining motor vehicle accidents are caused by drivers impaired by alcohol or drugs (Figs. 4-6, 4-7).

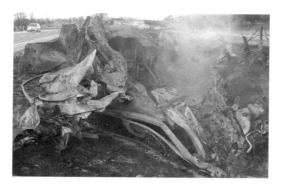
Figure 4-6: Motor vehicle of drunk driver after head-on collision and fire.

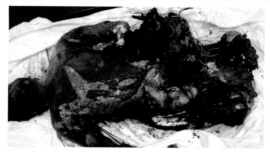
Figure 4-7: Body of drunk driver after motor vehicle accident with fire.

During 2005, 16,885 Americans died in alcohol-related motor vehicle accidents, constituting 39 percent of all traffic-related deaths (6). That year, 414 children ages fourteen and under died in alcohol-related auto crashes (6). Another forty-eight children in this age group were killed as pedestrians (Fig. 4-8) or as cyclists struck by alcohol-impaired drivers (6).

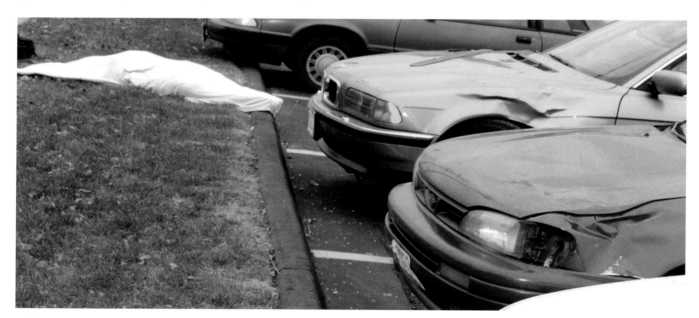
Figure 4-8: Body of a child hit by a motorist while walking on the sidewalk. Victim bounced off two parked cars before landing in grass.

One study estimated that there are 159 million self-reported episodes of alcohol-impaired driving among US adults each year (7). Drugs other than alcohol (but often used in combination with alcohol) are involved in approximately 18 percent of motor vehicle deaths (8).

Other factors associated with motor vehicle accidents are speeding, aggressive driving, and inexperience. Per mile driven, teenagers are four times more likely to crash than adult drivers. Drivers over age seventy-five also have an increased accident rate.

RECOMMENDATIONS FOR DECREASING YOUR RISK OF TRAFFIC ACCIDENTS

1. Focus on driving rather than multitasking.
2. Never text while on the road.
3. Don't drive when you are drowsy.
4. Don't drive when you have used alcohol or drugs. While most states consider a blood alcohol concentration (BAC) level of 0.08 to mean that a person is legally intoxicated, driving impairment begins at a much lower concentration. Some have estimated that a person with a BAC of 0.08 is eleven times more likely to be in an accident than a nondrinker, while a BAC of 0.05 doubles your accident risk. A 100-pound woman can obtain a BAC of 0.05 after only one drink. Don't risk driving after you have been drinking. The only safe BAC is 0.

POISONING

A poison is defined as any substance that is harmful to your body when eaten, inhaled, injected, or absorbed through the skin (12). Almost any substance can be poisonous if consumed in large enough quantities. Each day in the United States, unintentional poisoning causes nearly two thousand emergency room visits and seventy-five deaths (12).

Over 90 percent of unintentional poisoning deaths are caused by drugs (12). The accidental drug poisoning death rate has been rising, and more than doubled between 1999 and 2006 (13). In adults and older children, these deaths are often caused when overdosing on a drug abused for recreational purposes or otherwise not taken as prescribed. Younger children may ingest the medications of others if they gain access to these drugs while unsupervised. Other causes of poisoning include ingestion or exposure to household chemicals or carbon monoxide.

RECOMMENDATIONS FOR DECREASING YOUR RISK OF POISONING (14)

1. Don't abuse drugs.
2. Read all warning labels on medications, cleaning supplies, and chemicals.
3. Take medications only as directed.
4. Keep medicines in their original containers.
5. Keep medications in a safe place that cannot be reached by small children.
6. Properly dispose of unneeded or expired drugs.
7. Keep chemical products in their original containers, and never store them in used food containers.
8. Never mix household chemicals. For example, mixing bleach and ammonia can result in toxic gases.
9. Wear protective clothing if you spray chemicals or pesticides.
10. Allow good ventilation such as a ceiling fan or an open window when using chemical products.
11. Make sure all gas appliances and fireplaces are properly vented and serviced.
12. Never use a charcoal barbecue grill, portable gas camp stove, or gas-powered generator indoors.
13. Never run an automobile with the garage door shut.
14. Have the exhaust system of your car regularly checked for leaks.
15. Store household chemicals out of reach of small children.

16. Never leave children alone with household chemicals or drugs.
17. Don't call medicine "candy" around small children.
18. Try to avoid taking medications in front of small children, as they may try to copy your behavior.

IF POISONING OCCURS:

1. Try to remain calm.
2. If you or the victim has collapsed, call 9-1-1.
3. Assuming you or the victim is awake and alert, call the national poison control number at 1-800-222-1222.

FALLS

Injuries from falls are most frequent among the elderly and children. Among adults age sixty-five and older, falls are the most common cause of accident-related death (10). More than one-third of adults in this age group fall each year, resulting in over 15,000 deaths, 1.8 million emergency room visits, 433,000 hospitalizations, and over $19 billion in medical costs (10). The most common serious injuries from falls are head trauma and bone fractures. The risk of serious injury as a result of falling increases with age. Nearly 85 percent of fall-related deaths occur in people older than seventy-five (10).

RECOMMENDATIONS TO PREVENT OLDER ADULTS FROM FALLING (10)

1. Exercise regularly to increase strength and improve balance.
2. Review medications with your doctor or pharmacist to reduce side effects and interactions.
3. Have an eye exam at least once a year.
4. Improve lighting in the home. Open blinds to let sunshine in during the day. Use adequate lights at night.
5. Reduce hazards in the home that could lead to falls. Have snow and ice cleared from sidewalks. Use rubber mats in slick bathtubs. Don't let electrical cords lie over walkways.

Falls are also the most common cause of nonfatal injury of children in the United States (11). Each year, about 2.8 million children are admitted to emergency rooms for fall-related injuries (11).

RECOMMENDATIONS TO PREVENT CHILDREN FROM FALLING (11)

1. Make play areas safe. Check equipment for proper design, and provide a soft landing surface below.
2. Make home safety improvements including guards on all windows, gates on all staircases, and guardrails on the child's bed.
3. Make sure children wear protective gear such as knee pads, elbow pads, wrist guards, and helmets when playing potentially hazardous sports.
4. Supervise young children at all times around fall hazards such as stairs and playground equipment.

FIRES

According to United States Fire Statistics (15):

1. Fires injure someone every 31 minutes (Fig. 4-9).
2. Fires kill someone every 158 minutes.
3. Eighty percent of fire deaths occur in homes.
4. Firefighters respond to over 400,000 home fires every year.

5. Most fire victims die from smoke or poisonous gas rather than from burns.
6. Smoking is the leading cause of fire-related death.
7. Cooking is the leading cause of residential fires.
8. Alcohol use contributes to 40 percent of residential fire deaths.

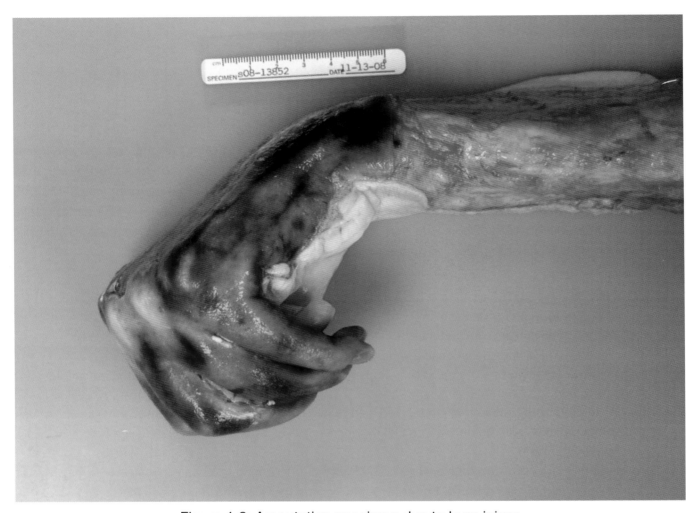

Figure 4-9: Amputation specimen due to burn injury.

RECOMMENDATIONS FOR FIRE PREVENTION AND SAFETY (16, 17, 18)

1. **Quit smoking.** If causing atherosclerosis, cancer, and COPD isn't bad enough, smoking is also the leading cause of fire death. If you do smoke, smoke outside. If you must smoke inside your home, at least don't smoke in bed, while you are drinking, or if you are overly tired. Never smoke around flammable liquids such as gasoline or cleaning fluids, and never smoke in a home where oxygen tanks are in use. Use large, deep ashtrays, and wet the ashes and cigarette butts before putting them in the trash.

2. **Be careful when cooking.** Don't leave the kitchen when frying, grilling, or broiling food. If you must leave, turn off the heat. Keep anything that can catch fire away from the stove top. Wipe up spilled grease. Don't pour water on a grease fire; rather, turn off the stove and cover the pan with a lid, or close the oven door. Keep a multipurpose ABC-type fire extinguisher in the kitchen. And don't cook when you have been drinking or are overly tired.

3. **Monitor children at all times.** Twenty-five percent of children's deaths caused by fires are fires started

by children. Keep lighters and matches out of their reach, and maintain a three-foot "kid-free zone" around stoves, fireplaces, and space heaters.

4. **Don't underestimate the clothes dryer.** Clean the lint screen frequently, as lint is highly flammable. Make sure the dryer is vented to the outside rather than a wall or attic.

5. **Properly store all flammable liquids.** Store these materials only in approved containers. Gas up equipment outside, away from sparks and heat. Start equipment at least ten feet from where it was filled with fuel. Don't fuel up lawn mowers or other equipment when they are hot, and never use gasoline as a cleaning fluid.

6. **Beware of electric hazards.** Don't overload sockets or use equipment with frayed or worn cords. If you see signs of electrical overload, such as lights that dim when an appliance goes on, a shrinking TV picture, slow appliance function, or frequent blown fuses, call an electrician. Allow air space around electrical appliances to prevent overheating. Don't use lightbulbs with wattage too high for the fixture—remember, the labels on each fixture list the maximum wattage. Check for loose wires or wall receptacles, and never run electric cords under a rug.

7. **Use space heaters with caution.** Maintain and inspect all heating equipment, including furnaces and space heaters. Turn off portable heaters before leaving the room or going to bed. Keep space heaters at least three feet from anything that could burn. Don't store anything flammable near a furnace or hot water heater.

8. **Keep an eye on candles and fireplaces.** Blow out candles before leaving the room or going to sleep. Use a fireplace screen on every fireplace in your home, and have your chimney inspected annually for creosote buildup.

9. **Install smoke detectors.** You should have a smoke detector in every bedroom, outside each sleeping area, and on every level of the home. Test smoke alarms every month to make sure they don't need a new battery.

10. **Know your exit plan.** Have a family fire exit plan with at least two ways out of each room. If a closed door feels hot, don't open it—take another path instead. Keep exit paths free of obstructions, and agree on a location outdoors where all occupants will meet for a head count. Don't return to a burning building. Stay together and call 9-1-1 from a safe location.

DROWNING

About ten people drown each day in the United States (19). More than 20 percent of drowning victims are younger than fourteen years old, and drowning is second only to motor vehicle accidents as a cause of accidental death among children (19). For every child that drowns, four receive medical care for nonfatal submersion injuries. These injuries can result in brain damage leading to memory problems, learning disabilities, or a permanent vegetative state (19). The most common sites of drowning vary with age. Infants younger than one year of age most frequently drown in bathtubs, buckets, or toilets (19). Children between ages one and fifteen typically drown in swimming pools, whereas drowning deaths among children older than age fifteen usually occur in natural bodies of water (19).

RECOMMENDATIONS FOR DECREASING THE RISK OF DROWNING (19)

1. **Supervise children closely.** Most young children who have drowned were in the care of a parent and were reported to be out of sight for less than five minutes (19). Pool fences with self-closing doors can help prevent children from entering the pool without their caregivers' knowledge. It is recommended that supervisors of preschool children be close enough to touch them at all times (19). Don't be involved with other distracting activities when supervising children around water.

2. **Wear life jackets.** Most boating accidental deaths are caused by drowning; 90 percent of the drowning

victims associated with boating accidents were not wearing life jackets (19). Do not use air-filled or foam toys such as water wings, noodles, or inner tubes in place of life jackets.

3. **Avoid alcohol when in or around water.** Alcohol impairs judgment, balance, and coordination, and is involved in nearly 50 percent of adolescent and adult deaths associated with water recreation (19). For all these reasons, don't drink when you are supervising children, either.

4. **Teach your children to swim.** The drowning rate of children is inversely proportional to their ability to swim (19).

5. **Use the buddy system.** It's safer to swim with a buddy. Areas with lifeguards add another protective factor.

6. **Be careful around rough water.** Avoid swimming in dangerous waves and strong currents. If you find yourself caught under a strong current, don't fight it. Let it carry you until it subsides and then head for shore.

PERSONAL OBSERVATIONS

When my children were young, they were sometimes sorry that I was a pathologist. Many times they would ask to participate in some risky activity and I would say no. I would then tell them about how I had seen some mutilated body part that resulted from someone doing what they were asking to do. The illustrations in this chapter are graphic, but I hope that these images may help prevent accidental injury to your loved ones or yourself.

REFERENCES:

1. Heron M. "Deaths: Leading Causes for 2004." *National Vital Statistics Reports* 56, no. 5 (2007): 1–95.

2. US Census Bureau. "Deaths from Accidents, by Type." Statistical Abstract of the United States (1999): 106, table 146.

3. "The 6 Most Common Causes of Automobile Crashes." www.sixwise.com.

4. Centers for Disease Control and Prevention. "Motor Vehicle Safety." Atlanta, GA: CDC, April 26, 2010. http://www.cdc.gov/Motorvehiclesafety/.

5. National Highway Traffic Safety Administration. "Virginia Tech Transportation Institute Release Findings of Breakthrough Research on Real-World Driver Behavior, Distraction and Crash Factors." April 20, 2006. http://www.nhtsa.gov/Driving+Safety/Distracted+Driving+at+Distraction.gov/Breakthrough+Research+on+Real-World+Driver+Behavior+Released.

6. Department of Transportation (US), National Highway Traffic Safety Administration (NHTSA). "Traffic Safety Facts 2005: Alcohol." Washington, DC, 2006.

7. Quinlan et al. "Alcohol-Impaired Driving among US Adults, 1993–2002." *American Journal of Preventive Medicine* 28 (2005): 345–50.

8. Jones et al. "State of Knowledge of Drug-Impaired Driving." Department of Transportation (US),

National Highway Traffic Safety Administration (NHTSA). Washington, DC, 2003. Report DOT HS 809 642.

9. Ohayon MM. "The Comorbid Conditions of Excessive Sleepiness in the American Population." In abstract supplement, *Sleep* 33 (2010): A266.

10. Centers for Disease Control and Prevention. "Falls among Older Adults: An Overview." Atlanta, GA: CDC, October 6, 2009. http://www.cdc.gov/homeandrecreationalsafety/falls/adultfalls.html.

11. Centers for Disease Control and Prevention. "Falls: The Reality." Atlanta, GA: CDC, July 27, 2009. http://www.cdc.gov/safechild/Falls/.

12. Centers for Disease Control and Prevention. "Poisoning in the United States: Fact Sheet." Atlanta, GA: CDC, March 18, 2010. www.cdc.gov.

13. Centers for Disease Control and Prevention. "CDC's Issue Brief: Unintentional Drug Poisoning in the United States." Atlanta, GA: CDC, March 18, 2010. http://www.cdc.gov/homeandrecreationalsafety/pdf/poison-issue-brief.pdf.

14. Centers for Disease Control and Prevention. "Tips to Prevent Poisonings." Atlanta, GA: CDC, March 12, 2010. http://www.cdc.gov/HomeandRecreationalSafety/Poisoning/preventiontips.htm.

15. Centers for Disease Control and Prevention. "Fire Deaths and Injuries: Fact Sheet." Atlanta, GA: CDC, October 2, 2009. www.cdc.gov.

16. Sheehan MJ. "Fire Prevention in the Home." seniors.tcnet.org.

17. Hall JR. "The Smoking-Material Fire Problem." National Fire Protection Association. Quincy, MA, March 2010.

18. National Fire Protection Association. "NFPA Study: Nearly All Structure Fire Deaths Happen in Home Fires." NFPA news release. May 25, 2010. http://www.nfpa.org/press-room/news-releases/2010/nfpa-study-nearly-all-structure-fire-deaths-happen-in-home-fires.

19. Centers for Disease Control and Prevention. "Unintentional Drowning: Fact Sheet." Atlanta, GA: CDC, June 7, 2010. http://www.cdc.gov/HomeandRecreationalSafety/Water-Safety/waterinjuries-factsheet.html.

5: DIABETES

Diabetes is not a single disease, but rather a group of disorders associated with hyperglycemia, or high blood glucose levels. Diabetes affects an estimated 16 million people in the United States and more than 140 million people worldwide. It is the leading cause of end-stage kidney disease, adult-onset blindness, and non-traumatic leg amputations in the United States. Each year in the US, approximately 800,000 people develop diabetes, and over 50,000 die of the disease. The estimated lifetime risk of being diagnosed with diabetes in the United States is one in three for males, and two in five for females; the risk is even higher in African American, Hispanic, and Native American populations. The number of people diagnosed with diabetes is expected to double—double!—by the year 2025 (1).

BACKGROUND INFORMATION

Glucose is a simple sugar derived from food. Glucose intake and subsequent high blood levels of glucose stimulate the release of insulin, a hormone produced by the beta cells in the pancreas. Insulin promotes the uptake of glucose into skeletal muscle and fat. In muscle, the glucose is stored as glycogen, while in fat cells, the glucose is converted to lipid and stored as fat. When blood glucose levels drop between meals, glucagon is released from alpha cells in the pancreas. Glucagon stimulates the production of glucose from the liver and glycogen breakdown in muscle to keep blood glucose levels from falling too low. Normally blood glucose levels are maintained between 70 and 120 mg/dl (1). If the blood glucose is too low, you may experience hunger, headache, weakness, nervousness, trembling, or sweating. High blood glucose levels can lead to thirst, frequent urination, difficulty concentrating, and fatigue.

PATHOLOGY

The diagnosis of diabetes occurs when a patient demonstrates hyperglycemia according to one of these three criteria (1):

1. A random blood glucose level of greater than 200 mg/dl with signs and symptoms of the disease, such as chronic thirst and frequent urination.
2. A fasting glucose level greater than 126 mg/dl on more than one occasion.
3. An abnormal glucose tolerance test in which glucose is greater than 200 mg/dl two hours after drinking a solution with 75 grams of glucose.

There are two major categories of diabetes:

- Type 1 diabetes (which constitutes 10 percent of all cases) is caused by a deficiency of insulin due to the destruction of beta cells in the pancreas.
- Type 2 diabetes (constituting the remaining 90 percent of all cases) is caused by insulin resistance of target tissues such as muscle, fat, and the liver.

Type 1 diabetes commonly develops in childhood. It is an autoimmune disease in which our immune system attacks and destroys beta cells in the pancreas.

The autoimmune reaction in type 1 diabetes may be predisposed by genetic factors. There is also evidence that environmental factors, especially viral infections, may contribute to the disease. Viruses likely don't destroy pancreatic beta cells directly; rather, most evidence suggests that infection may induce tissue damage with the release of beta-cell antigens, which attract the attention of the immune system. A second theory proposes that the viruses themselves produce proteins that mimic targets on beta cells. The resulting immune response to these proteins may cross-react with the insulin-producing cells in the pancreas (1). Whatever the mechanism, in type 1 diabetes the body's immune system attacks and destroys the cells in the pancreas that produce insulin.

Insulin resistance is one of the key elements of type 2 diabetes. In this condition, insulin is not effective in stimulating glucose uptake by muscle and fat cells. Insulin in these patients also fails to suppress hepatic glucose production. Patients with type 2 diabetes have normal levels of functional insulin. The problem lies in the target tissues; namely, the muscle, fat, and liver. Abnormalities including decreased insulin receptors and decreased cellular activity in the insulin-signaling pathway—in other words, insulin still turns the key, but the cellular machinery doesn't start—have been found in this condition.

Insulin resistance is closely linked with obesity, and the risk of type 2 diabetes increases as a person's body fat increases (1). Patients whose fat is predominantly found in their abdominal area are especially prone to this disease. Just how obesity causes insulin resistance is not fully understood. Increased circulating fat in the bloodstream, increased intracellular fat, and hormones released by fat cells (adipokines) are thought to contribute to insulin resistance (1). Another reason (besides the threat of atherosclerosis, cancer, and fatty liver disease) to keep your weight under control!

Beta-cell dysfunction is another aspect of type 2 diabetes. Early in the disease, type 2 diabetic patients show high insulin levels in an attempt to compensate for the insulin resistance. However, over time, beta cells fail to overcompensate for the peripheral insulin resistance. The reason for the beta-cell failure at this stage of the disease is not well understood. It has been proposed that the high amounts of circulating fats and sugar in the bloodstream may have toxic effects on beta cells (1).

Chronic hyperglycemia associated with diabetes takes its toll on many parts of the body. The most prominent changes are seen in the patient's arteries, small vessels, kidneys, retinas, and nerves.

Diabetic arterial disease: Diabetes accelerates the development of atherosclerosis of large arteries (see chapter 1). Heart attacks are the most common cause of death in diabetics. Gangrene of the lower extremities (Figs. 5-1A to 5-1C) is about 100 times more common in diabetics than in nondiabetics.

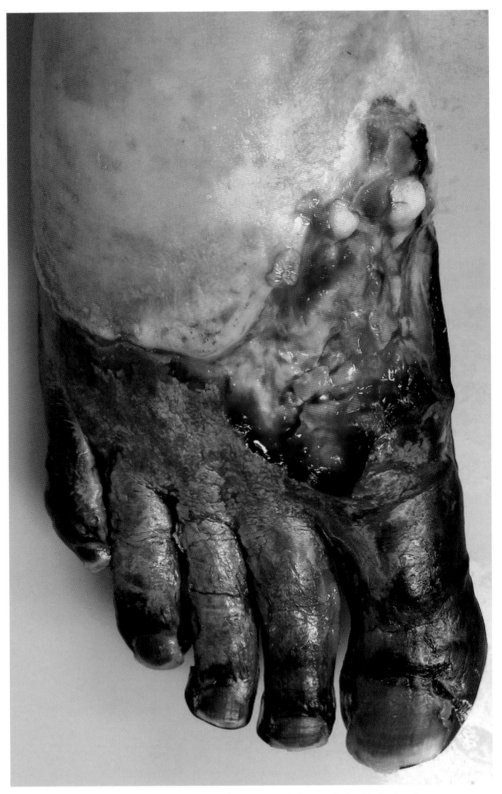

Figure 5-1A: Necrosis (gangrene) in a diabetic's foot.

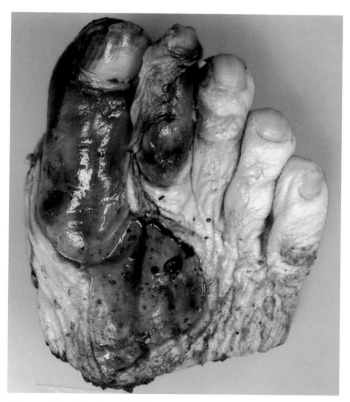

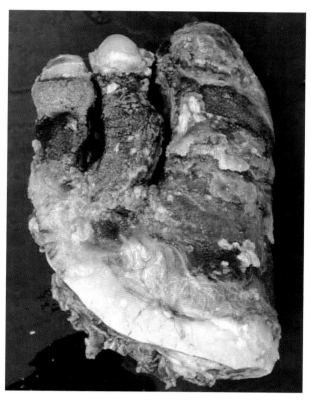

Figure 5-1B: Partial foot amputation for gangrene.   Figure 5-1C: Gangrene.

Diabetes also causes the thickening of the walls of small arteries, which further decreases the blood flow to many cells in the body (Figs. 5-2A, 5-2B).

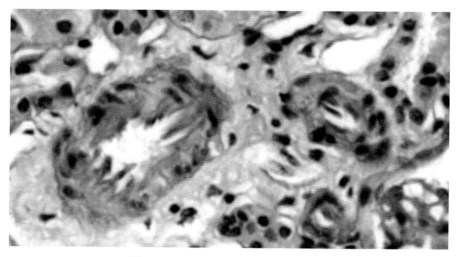

Figure 5-2A: Normal arterioles.

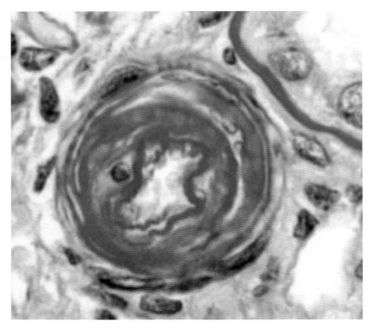

Figure 5-2B: Diabetic arteriolosclerosis.

Diabetic nephropathy: Our kidneys have millions of glomeruli, which act as tiny filters that remove waste from our blood while retaining vital blood components. In chronic diabetes, the glomeruli are damaged (Figs. 5-3A, 5-3B).

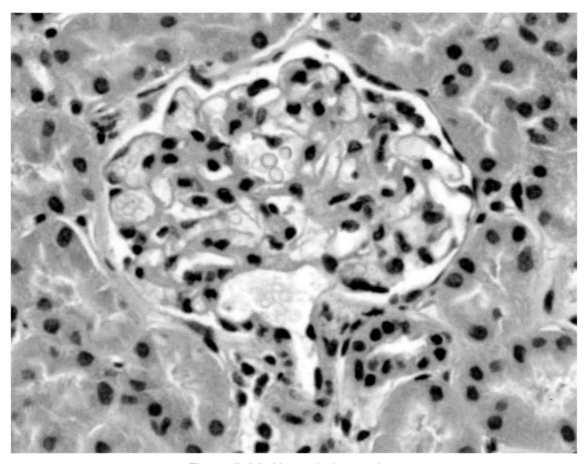

Figure 5-3A: Normal glomerulus.

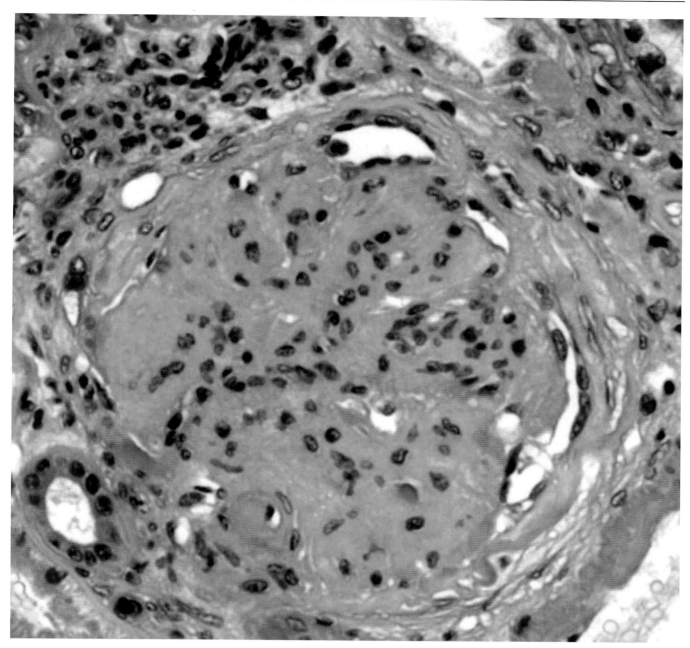

Figure 5-3B: Diabetic glomerulosclerosis.

The damaged glomeruli become leaky and lose the proteins usually retained in the blood. Eventually, the glomeruli become nonfunctional, resulting in renal failure (Fig. 5-3C).

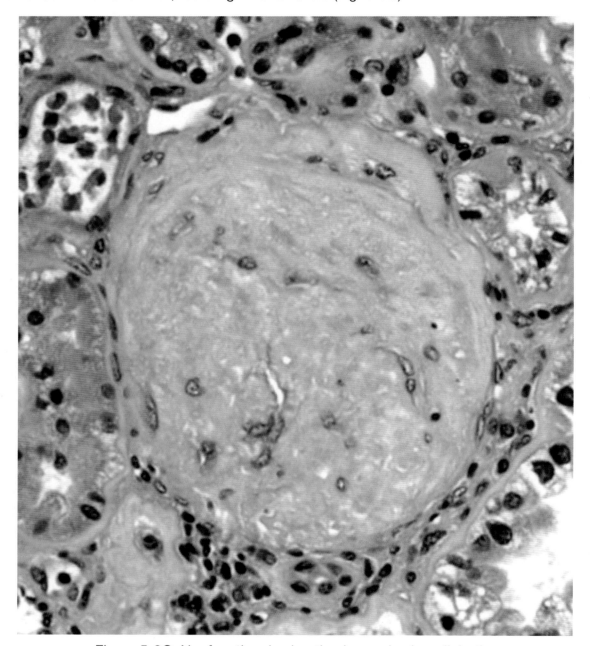

Figure 5-3C: Nonfunctional sclerotic glomerulus in a diabetic.

The high blood sugar levels in diabetics also hamper the ability of white blood cells to fight infections, leading to increased kidney infections.

      Ocular complications: Diabetes causes multiple eye problems, including cataract formation (when the lens becomes cloudy), glaucoma (when the eye experiences increased pressure, with damage to the optic nerve), and diabetic retinopathy. Diabetic retinopathy is the most serious eye-related complication of diabetes. The retina functions as a camera to collect visual images, which are then sent to the brain. Retinal blood vessels, like other small vessels, become thickened in diabetics. Damage to these small retinal vessels leads to poor blood supply to the retina. This stimulates the proliferation of new vessels, which can block light transmission to the optic disc and retina, leading to blindness.

Diabetic neuropathy: Approximately half of long-term diabetic patients have clinical signs of nerve damage. Vessels feeding nerves show the same thickening as other small vessels. The thickened vessels decrease the blood supply and cause damage to the nerve. Diabetic patients with nerve damage may lose the ability to sense pain. Because of this they do not know when minor trauma or pressure is leading to tissue damage. This can result in ulcers (Fig. 5-4). The ulcers tend to heal poorly because of the vascular damage in diabetics.

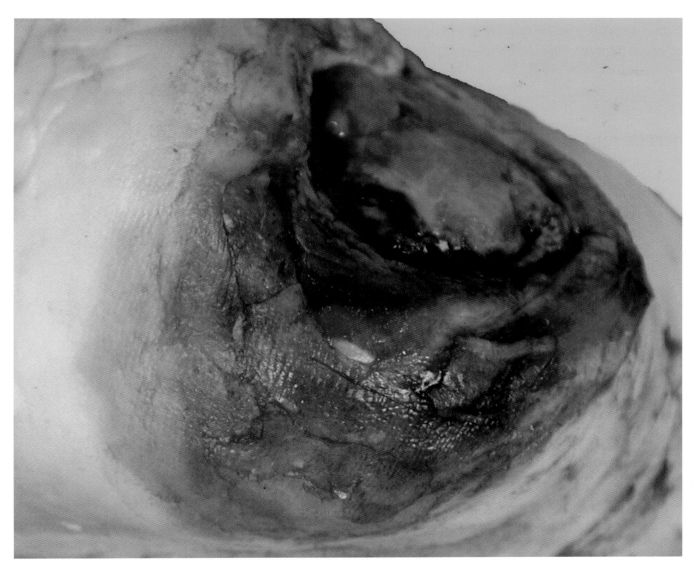

Figure 5-4: Diabetic ulcer on heel leading to foot amputation.

Infection: By damaging blood vessels and making the body's immune cells less functional, the hyperglycemia associated with diabetes results in increased susceptibility to infections. Infections ultimately result in death for about 5 percent of diabetic patients.

RISK FACTORS

Type 2 diabetes is closely associated with a sedentary lifestyle and obesity. Studies have shown that lifestyle changes, such as adding thirty minutes of moderate exercise five times per week and avoiding being overweight, could prevent, or at least delay, most cases of type 2 diabetes (2). Vitamin D supplements may decrease the incidence of both types of diabetes (3).

PERSONAL OBSERVATIONS

Diabetes is a common disease that causes much suffering and many deaths. I've seen this disease cause many cases of gangrene, kidney failure, and heart attacks. The incidence of type 2 diabetes continues to rise with the rising incidence of obesity. Fortunately, most cases of type 2 diabetes can be prevented by moderate exercise and weight control. These relatively simple lifestyle choices could decrease the incidence of this terrible disease by nearly 90 percent.

REFERENCES:

1. Maitra A, Abbas AK. "The Endocrine System." In *Robbins and Cotran Pathologic Basis of Disease*, 7th ed., edited by Kumar et al, 1189–1205. Philadelphia, PA: Elsevier Saunders, 2005.

2. Chiasson JL. "Prevention of Type 2 Diabetes: Fact or Fiction?" *Expert Opinion on Pharmacotherapy* 8, no. 18 (2007): 3147–58.

3. Danescu et al. "Vitamin D and Diabetes Mellitus." *Endocrine Reviews* 35 (2009): 11–17.

6: CIRRHOSIS

Cirrhosis is a major cause of death in the Western world, killing about twenty-six thousand US citizens each year (1). A result of chronic liver injury, cirrhosis is most commonly due to ingested toxins such as alcohol; viruses, including hepatitis B and C; and metabolic derangements, like fatty liver disease associated with obesity (2).

BACKGROUND INFORMATION

At approximately three pounds, the liver is the largest gland in the body. It has many diverse functions, including the metabolism of amino acids, carbohydrates, and hormones; the production of numerous proteins; the regulation of lipid and cholesterol metabolism; and the breakdown of the drugs and toxins we ingest (3). The liver is the only internal organ with the capability to significantly regenerate. Within a few weeks, the liver can grow back to its normal size after the surgical excision of over half its mass!

PATHOLOGY

Despite the liver's amazing regenerative capacity, chronic liver injury can overwhelm its ability to heal itself and can cause liver failure. Chronic liver damage, like that seen in alcohol abuse or chronic viral hepatitis, can cause scarring of the liver. Damaged liver cells try to regenerate but are trapped in the scar tissue and form nodules of liver tissue that do not have normal circulation. The term "cirrhosis" is used for this end-stage liver disease. Cirrhosis often leads to death through progressive liver failure, increased blood pressure in the blood vessels draining into the liver, or the development of a liver cancer called hepatocellular carcinoma (Figs. 6-1A, 6-1B).

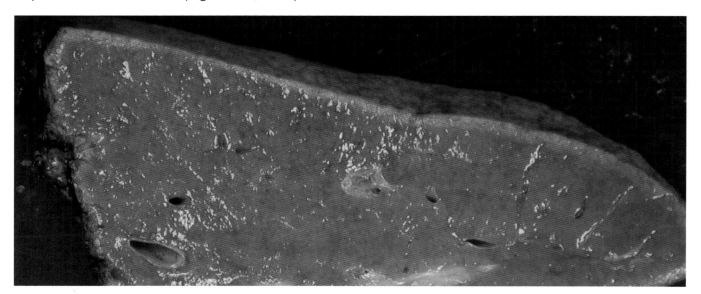

Figure 6-1A: Cut surface of a relatively normal liver.

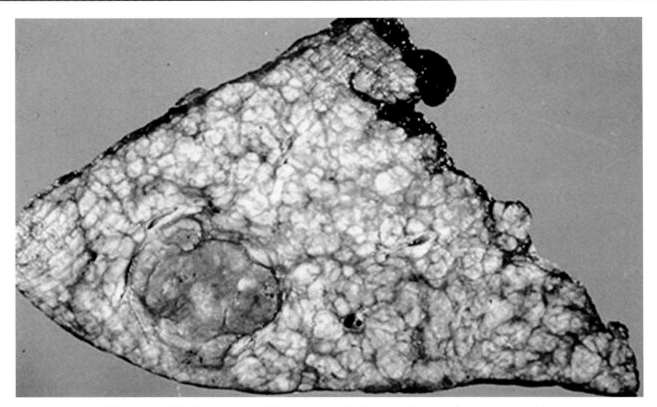

Figure 6-1B: Cirrhosis with hepatocellular carcinoma (green nodule).
Photo courtesy of Alberto Diaz-Arias, MD.

The scarring in cirrhosis leads to decreased blood flow to liver cells and the obstruction of the channels through which bile flows. Thus, the liver's ability to filter the blood and deliver the proteins it produces is severely compromised. Obstruction of the flow of bile leads to jaundice, which causes a yellow discoloration of the eyes and skin.

Deteriorating liver function is associated with increased blood levels of substances normally filtered out by the liver. Increased blood levels of toxic substances like ammonia are associated with changes in brain function. These changes, called hepatic encephalopathy, can cause behavioral abnormalities, confusion, stupor, coma, and death (2).

Cirrhosis increases the resistance of blood flow through the liver. This causes many problems. Blood backs up into the portal vein, a large vein that drains into the liver. Congestion in the portal vein leads to congestion of organs and vessels that drain into it. This results in enlargement of the spleen, congestion of vessels around the anus, and congestion of vessels in the esophagus (the tube that transports food from your mouth to your stomach). The enlarged, congested spleen tends to filter out components of the blood that normally pass through it. For example, normal platelets in the blood, which help blood clot, can be removed, causing bleeding problems. Congestion of blood vessels around the anus causes hemorrhoids, which can be an irritating source of bleeding and discomfort. Congested vessels in the esophagus, called esophageal varices, are more serious. When they rupture, they often cause fatal hemorrhage (2).

Hepatocellular carcinoma, a cancer of liver cells (Fig. 6-2), is closely associated with chronic liver damage and cirrhosis.

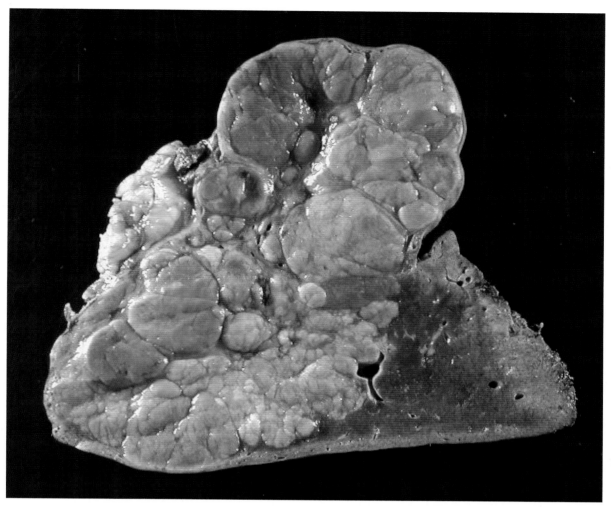

Figure 6-2: Hepatocellular carcinoma extensively replacing liver.

The incidence of hepatocellular carcinoma in North America is about five cases per one hundred thousand people. In parts of Asia and Africa where hepatitis B is more widespread, the incidence approaches thirty-six cases per one hundred thousand people; in some of these areas, it is the most common type of cancer (2). In the US, about 90 percent of these tumors develop in patients with cirrhosis (2). Hepatocellular carcinoma is an especially serious cancer; if left untreated, the median time of survival is approximately four months. Even with treatment, the overall five-year survival rate in the United States is only 3 percent (4).

RISK FACTORS

Sadly, most cirrhosis-related deaths are due to poor lifestyle choices. In the United States, 60 to 70 percent of cirrhosis is due to alcoholic liver disease (2). The amount of alcohol that can be consumed without serious liver injury varies greatly from person to person. This variation in tolerance to alcohol is not well understood. However, in general, women are more at risk than men, and African Americans are more at risk than white Americans. A family history of alcoholic liver disease, and the presence of other liver diseases such as viral hepatitis, also increase the risk of developing alcoholic liver damage. Though alcoholic cirrhosis typically develops after more than a decade of heavy drinking, cirrhosis can develop with as few as two to three drinks per day (1). (See chapter 8 for more information on the consequences of alcohol.)

Ten percent of cirrhosis in the US is caused by viral hepatitis, mainly hepatitis C and hepatitis B (2). These types of hepatitis are transferred in infected blood. About 75 percent of cases of hepatitis B and C are transmitted by intravenous drug use or through sexual intercourse (2). Many of the remaining cases are due to transfusion blood products—blood was not screened for hepatitis C prior to 1991—and health care provider accidents, such as a nurse or doctor sticking themselves with a needle removed from an infected patient. (2). In areas of Africa and Asia where hepatitis B is common, the virus commonly spreads from mother to child during childbirth (2).

In the United States, most of the remaining cases of cirrhosis are due to nonalcoholic fatty liver disease (NAFL), which is closely associated with obesity and type 2 diabetes (2). It is estimated that 31 million Americans have NAFL (2). Under the microscope, NAFL looks like alcoholic liver disease. The first noticeable change is the accumulation of fat in liver cells. Later, the fat may be associated with inflammation and fibrosis of the liver.

Studies suggest that 10 to 30 percent of patients with NAFL will eventually develop cirrhosis (2). Given the current epidemic of obesity in our country, there is a growing concern that NAFL will cause an increased number of cirrhosis cases in the near future. NAFL is treated with lifestyle modifications including diet and exercise (2). The changes do not have to be extreme to be effective. Gradual weight loss of 10 percent of your body weight, and sixty minutes of low-intensity exercise (such as walking) per week can reverse the disease.

PERSONAL OBSERVATIONS

As outlined in this chapter, most cases of cirrhosis in the USA are caused by alcohol, drug abuse, high-risk sexual behavior, or obesity. The good news is that the most common causes of cirrhosis can be avoided with lifestyle choices. One of the patients from medical school that I remember most vividly was a thirty-one-year-old man with advanced cirrhosis due to alcohol abuse. He had overcome his addiction to alcohol, but the liver damage was so severe that he knew he would soon die and leave his family. It was a tragic situation. Don't let this happen to you!

REFERENCES:

1. National Institute of Diabetes and Digestive and Kidney Diseases. "Cirrhosis of the Liver." NIH Publication No. 04-1134, December 2003.

2. Crawford JM. "Liver and Biliary Tract." In *Robbins and Cotran Pathologic Basis of Disease*, 7th ed., edited by Kumar et al, 837–937. Philadelphia, PA: Elsevier Saunders, 2005.

3. Podolsky DK, Isselbacher KJ. "Derangements of Hepatic Metabolism." In *Harrison's Principles of Internal Medicine*, 14th ed., edited by Fauci et al, 1667. New York, NY: McGraw-Hill, 1998.

4. Rosai J. *Rosai and Ackerman's Surgical Pathology*. 9th ed. St. Louis, MO: Mosby, 2004: 1002–03.

PART II
HIGH-RISK LIFESTYLE CHOICES

7: TOBACCO

Tobacco use, particularly cigarette smoking, is the world's leading cause of preventable disease and death (Fig. 7-1).

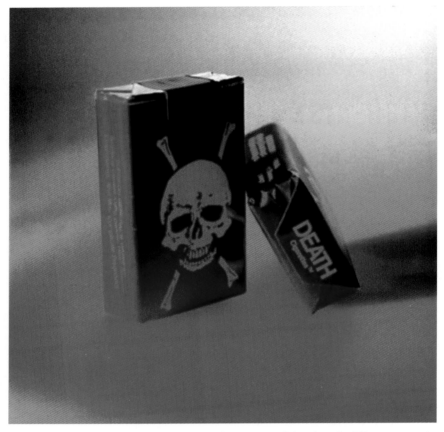

Figure 7-1: Smoking is the world's leading cause of preventable death. Photo courtesy of Bill Branson, National Cancer Institute.

Smoking is a major risk factor for the three leading causes of death in the United States: atherosclerosis, cancer, and chronic obstructive lung disease.

The damage to the human race as a result of cigarette smoking is staggering.

Consider the following statistics:

- Tobacco smoking killed 100 million people worldwide in the twentieth century. It is estimated that smoking may kill 1 billion people in the twenty-first century (1).
- Every eight seconds, someone dies from tobacco use (2).
- Tobacco kills approximately 440,000 US citizens each year, which equates to 1,205 Americans per day (3).
- Smoking costs the US health care system $157 billion each year (3).
- Worldwide, about one-third of adult males smoke (2).
- Nearly one-half of male smokers will die from smoking (2).
- It has been estimated that each cigarette shortens the smoker's life by five minutes (2).
- Approximately twelve times more British people have died from smoking than from World War II (2).

While smoking rates have been declining in the United States and in other developed countries, tobacco consumption is rising in the developing world, particularly in the Western Pacific Region.

A few more statistics:

- About two-thirds of Chinese men smoke cigarettes (2).
- Smoking kills 3,000 Chinese people every day (2).
- It is estimated that smoking will kill nearly one-third of all Chinese men under thirty years of age (2).
- Approximately 15 billion cigarettes are sold daily—that's 10 million per minute (2).
- Between 80,000 and 100,000 children start smoking every day (2).
- More than 4,000 different substances have been detected in cigarette smoke, including over fifty known carcinogens and substances such as hydrogen cyanide (the substance used in gas chamber executions), carbon monoxide (the poisonous gas found in car exhaust), formaldehyde (used as an embalming fluid), arsenic (used in rat poison), polonium-210 (a radioactive substance), and nicotine (3, 4).
- Smoking harms nearly every organ in the body (4).
- Of the 440,000 premature US deaths caused by smoking each year, about 40 percent are from cancer, 35 percent are from atherosclerosis, and 25 percent are from chronic lung disease (4) (Fig. 7-2).

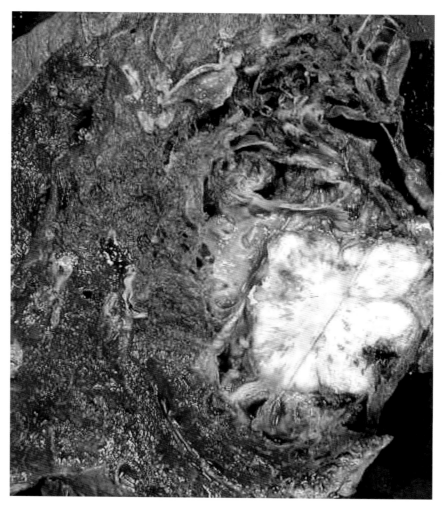

Figure 7-2: Smoker's lung showing emphysema (upper right) and cancer (lower right).

Smoking is the leading cause of cancer, causing 30 percent of all cancer deaths (3). It causes tumors of the lung, esophagus, larynx, mouth, throat, kidney, bladder, pancreas, stomach, and cervix (4). It is also involved in acute myeloid leukemia, a cancer of white blood cells (4). Evidence is mounting that smoking also contributes to other cancers, such as colon cancer and breast cancer.

Smoking is second only to high blood levels of cholesterol as a risk factor for atherosclerosis (5). The risk of dying from a heart attack is at least doubled in smokers compared to nonsmokers with the same age, blood pressure, and cholesterol levels (5). Smoking increases the formation of atherosclerosis by increasing low-density lipoproteins (LDLs), decreasing high-density lipoproteins (HDLs), increasing the oxidation of lipoproteins, increasing triglycerides, damaging endothelium, and increasing blood clots in arteries (5).

As outlined in chapter 3, smoking also causes about 90 percent of chronic obstructive pulmonary disease. Smoking contributes to many other diseases including pneumonia, weak bones with subsequent hip fractures, and cataracts (4). Other consequences of smoking include stained teeth and fingers, increased wrinkles, poor sleep quality, and decreased sexual performance.

Smoking also injures innocent bystanders. Each year, approximately 3,000 American nonsmokers die from lung cancer as a result of secondhand smoke, while 150,000 to 300,000 US infants develop smoke-related respiratory infections (6). Passive smoke exposure is a risk factor for childhood asthma and worsens the condition in up to 1 million American children (6). A pregnant smoker increases her baby's risk of low birth weight, premature birth, and sudden infant death syndrome, and exposure to smoke after the birth also increases an infant's risk of SIDS (4).

The nicotine in cigarette smoke is a highly addictive chemical. Some have concluded that it is more addictive than marijuana, caffeine, ethanol, cocaine, and heroin (7). Nicotine addiction occurs rapidly. A study of adolescents found signs of addiction began soon after the first puff; mental addiction was present after 2.5 months, cigarette cravings after 4.5 months, and physical addiction after 5.4 months (8). Most smokers become addicted to tobacco before they are old enough to legally buy cigarettes (9). Peer pressure, along with the constant images of smoking movie stars, are cited as reasons that many young people start smoking.

Once addicted to smoking, it is very difficult to stop. Indeed, it is much easier to never begin in the first place. With that said, the rewards of quitting smoking are well worth the effort required. People who quit smoking, regardless of their age, reduce their risk of dying from smoking-related diseases (4). For example, it is estimated that the risk of dying from a heart attack or stroke decreases 50 percent after one year of smoking cessation. Quitting sooner is better than later, as your risk for developing a smoking-related disease increases with each year spent smoking (4).

RECOMMENDATIONS FOR QUITTING SMOKING (4, 10)

1. **Convince yourself that you want and need to quit.** Rereading this chapter may be helpful. Pick a day to quit when stress will not be at a peak and stick to it.

2. **Talk with your doctor or pharmacist about medications that can help you quit smoking.** Popular medications include nicotine-replacement products, which can be purchased over the counter; Bupropion, a prescription antidepressant marketed as Zyban and Wellbutrin, which can reduce nicotine withdrawal symptoms as well as the urge to smoke; and Varenicline, a prescription medicine marketed as Chantix, which may ease withdrawal symptoms and block the effects of nicotine if smoking resumes.

3. **Seek help and support from family, friends, and free government resources.** Recommended resources include: SmokeFree.gov, a website established by the National Cancer Institute, which has many helpful resources to help you quit smoking, including publications and toll-free hotlines with counseling services (1-800-QUITNOW). LiveHelp is another excellent resource from the National Cancer Institute, and has counselors that speak English and Spanish (1-877-44U-QUIT).

4. **Adopt other healthy lifestyle changes while you quit to help improve your mood and prevent weight gain.** Daily exercise, such as walking, a balanced diet with lots of water, and plenty of sleep can be helpful.

PERSONAL OBSERVATIONS

During my medical career, I have seen firsthand the tremendous damage induced by smoking. Lung cancer can transform a healthy-looking body into an emaciated corpse within a few months. A heart attack can kill someone at the peak of their career within a few minutes. Chronic lung disease can cause a person to gasp for air like a drowning man. In the twentieth century, smoking killed as many people as World Wars I and II combined. It is predicted that it will kill *1 billion* people in the twenty-first century. How can this self-inflicted plague be avoided? If you smoke, please stop. If you don't smoke, don't start!

REFERENCES:

1. The WHO Report on the Global Tobacco Epidemic, 2008.

2. World Health Organization Regional Office for the Western Pacific. "Smoking Statistics." May 27, 2002. http://www.wpro.who.int/mediacentre/factsheets/fs_20020528/en/.

3. Kane AB, Kumar V. "Environmental and Nutritional Pathology." In *Robbins and Cotran Pathologic Basis of Disease*, 7th ed., edited by Kumar et al, 419–21. Philadelphia, PA: Elsevier Saunders, 2005.

4. "Quitting Smoking: Why to Quit and How to Get Help." National Cancer Institute Factsheet. August 17, 2007.

5. Erhardt L. "Cigarette Smoking: An Undertreated Risk Factor for Cardiovascular Disease." *Atherosclerosis* 205 (2009): 23–32.

6. Environmental Protection Agency. "Setting the Record Straight: Secondhand Smoke Is a Preventable Health Risk." EPA Document Number 402-F-94-005, June 1994.

7. Hilts PJ, "Relative Addictiveness of Drugs," *New York Times*, August 2, 1994.

8. Gervais et al. "Milestones in the Natural Course of Onset of Cigarette Use among Adolescents." *Canadian Medical Association Journal* 175, no. 3 (August 1, 2006): 255–61.

9. Cokkinides et al. "Tobacco Control in the United States—Recent Progress and Opportunities." *CA: A Cancer Journal for Clinicians* 59 (2009): 352–65.

10. American Lung Association, news release, December 2008.

8: ALCOHOL

Ethyl alcohol, otherwise known as ethanol, is the most widely used and abused mind-altering substance in the world (Fig. 8-1).

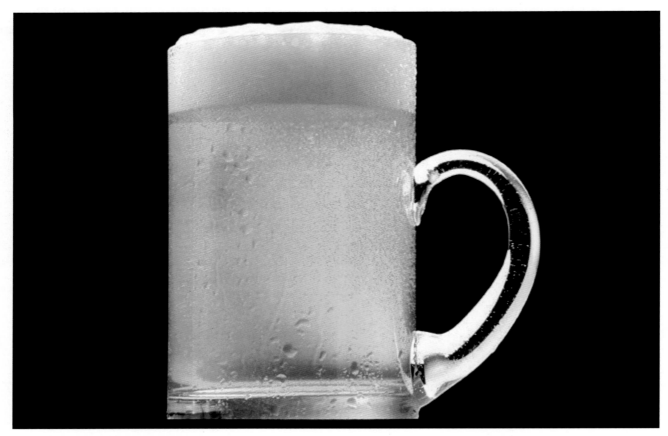

Figure 8-1: Alcohol is the world's most accepted and widely abused mind-altering substance. Photo courtesy of Len Rizzi, National Cancer Institute.

Each year, alcohol abuse kills approximately 200,000 people in the United States, with an economic cost of about $130 billion (1, 2). There are currently 15 to 20 million alcoholics in the US (1). Twenty-five to thirty percent of all hospitalized patients in the US have problems related to alcohol abuse (2). Obviously, this situation represents another great opportunity to prevent suffering through lifestyle changes.

SHORT-TERM EFFECTS OF DRINKING ALCOHOL
Alcohol is a potent central nervous system depressant with a wide range of effects depending on the blood alcohol concentration (BAC) level. Typical effects seen at different blood concentrations include (3, 5):

1. **Euphoria** (BAC of 0.03 to 0.12 percent): Improvement in mood along with possible euphoria. You may become more confident or daring. Judgment and fine motor movements are impaired. Even these relatively low blood alcohol levels are associated with significant effects. The US National Transportation Safety Board has calculated that driving with a BAC of 0.05 percent increases the risk of a traffic accident by 39 percent, and driving with a BAC of 0.08 percent increases the risk of a traffic accident by over 100 percent!
2. **Lethargy** (BAC of 0.09 to 0.25 percent): The drinker may become sleepy, body movements are uncoordinated, vision blurs, and reaction time is impaired.

3. **Confusion** (BAC of 0.18 to 0.30 percent): People are uncertain where they are or what they are doing. Dizziness, staggering, nausea, and vomiting may occur. The person may become overly emotional— either aggressive or affectionate.

4. **Stupor** (BAC of 0.25 to 0.40 percent): The person will lapse in and out of consciousness, may lose bladder control, and could have irregular breathing or heart rate. Risk of death due to alcoholic poisoning or aspiration of vomit.

5. **Coma** (BAC of 0.35 to 0.50 percent): Subject is unconscious with irregular breathing and heart rate. Death may occur.

6. **Death** (BAC of greater than 0.50 percent): Central nervous system failure results in death. A BAC of 0.55 percent will kill half of those affected.

It is important to note that alcohol has a relatively narrow safe active blood concentration. A BAC twice that of the level required to be drunk may turn out to be fatal (1). Fortunately, vomiting and extreme lethargy help prevent additional alcohol intake once one is intoxicated. Fatal blood alcohol concentrations are usually associated with a rapid ingestion of large amounts of concentrated alcoholic beverages. Unfortunately, this is often seen in young people as a result of drinking games or college initiation events, where as many as twenty alcoholic drinks are consumed in an hour.

OTHER SHORT-TERM EFFECTS OF DRINKING ALCOHOL:

- **Dehydration:** Alcohol decreases the production of antidiuretic hormone (ADH), the hormone that increases water reabsorption by the kidneys. Low ADH causes excessive urination, resulting in dehydration (3, 5).

- **Hangovers:** The day after intoxication, many experience symptoms of dry mouth, headache, nausea, and sensitivity to movement, light, and noise. These symptoms may be partly due to dehydration. Acetaldehyde, a toxic substance produced in the metabolism of alcohol, also contributes to hangovers (3, 5).

The impaired judgment and reaction time associated with alcohol use leads to many accidents, particularly motor vehicle accidents (Fig. 8-2). In the United States alone, alcohol-related motor vehicle crashes kill approximately 17,000 people per year (4).

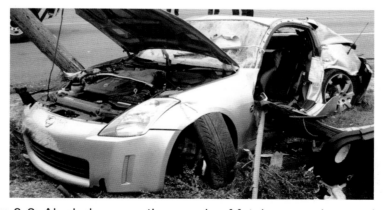

Figure 8-2: Alcohol causes thousands of fatal car crashes each year.

The impaired judgment and altered emotions associated with alcohol abuse can lead to behavior that could have been avoided had the person been sober. Physical injuries, drowning, jail sentences, sexually transmitted diseases, and unwanted pregnancies can all result from irresponsible drinking.

On an average day in the United States, alcohol is involved in: (5)
- The death of four college students
- The sexual assault of 192 college students
- The injury of 1,370 college students
- The assault of 1,644 college students

Annually in the United States, alcohol is involved in: (5)
- 25 percent of all emergency room visits
- 33 percent of all suicides
- 50 percent of all homicides
- 50 percent of all domestic violence incidents
- 50 percent of all traffic fatalities
- 50 percent of all fire fatalities

In addition, alcoholics have a divorce or separation rate at least four times greater than the general population (6).

LONG-TERM EFFECTS OF DRINKING ALCOHOL

In addition to the short-term effects of alcohol already listed, habitual drinking can have many more subtle effects on the body. Some of the most common changes follow.

Liver injury: Alcohol is metabolized by the liver. Both ethanol and its metabolic breakdown products are directly toxic to liver cells. The first and most common change seen in the liver is steatosis, where the liver is enlarged and yellow due to fat accumulation in liver cells (Fig. 8-3).

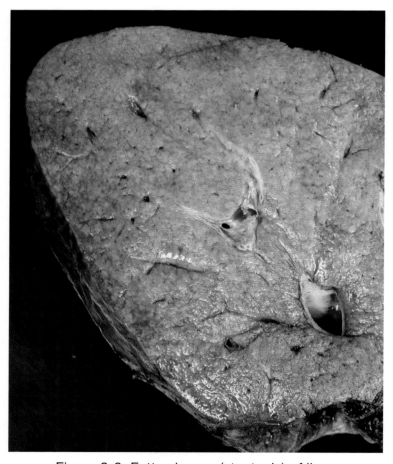

Figure 8-3: Fatty change (steatosis) of liver.

Steatosis usually does not cause symptoms. However, steatohepatitis, the next phase of liver injury, is associated with fever, tenderness, and jaundice. In this phase, dead liver cells and inflammation are seen (Figs. 8-4A, 8-4B).

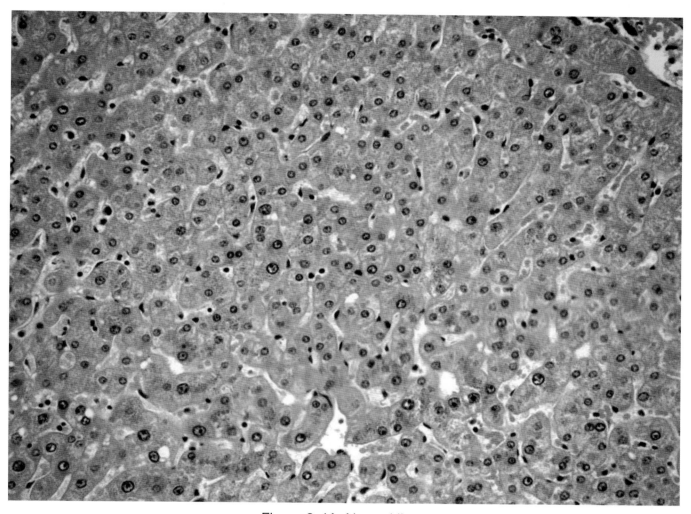

Figure 8-4A: Normal liver.

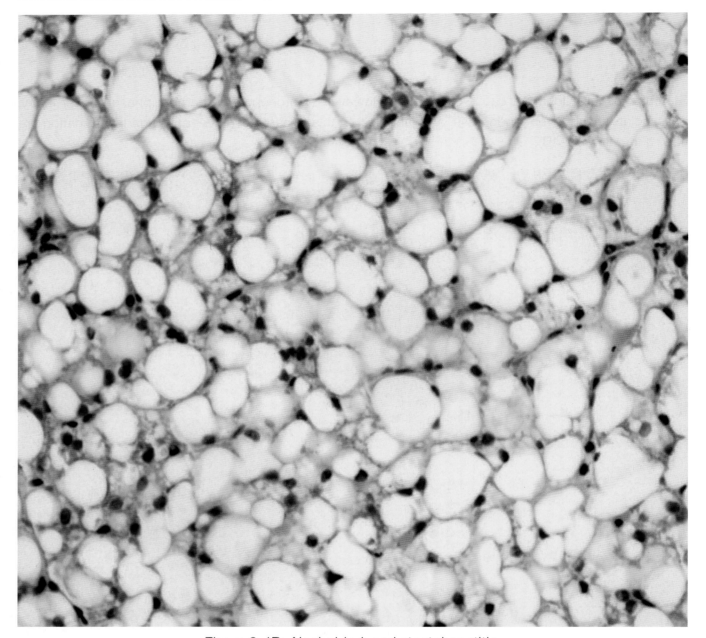

Figure 8-4B: Alcohol-induced steatohepatitis.

Ongoing steatohepatitis can lead to hepatic fibrosis and eventually cirrhosis. As described in chapter 6, cirrhosis is a potentially fatal disease accompanied by weakness, the wasting away of muscle, fluid collections in the abdomen, varices (distended veins of the esophagus), and hemorrhoids. Bleeding varices can cause fatal hemorrhage. Liver failure due to cirrhosis can lead to coma and death (1, 2).

Effects on cardiovascular system: Light chronic alcohol consumption, defined as one to two drinks per day, may increase high-density lipoproteins and help defend the body against atherosclerosis and ischemic heart disease. Heavier drinking is associated with direct damage to the heart muscle, or alcoholic cardiomyopathy. Chronic alcoholics commonly develop high blood pressure, which increases the risk of atherosclerosis (1, 5).

Effects on nervous system: Alcoholics tend to have poor nutrition, as a large percentage of their caloric intake typically comes from alcoholic beverages. Alcohol increases the body's requirements for the B vitamins and interferes with the absorption of thiamine from the intestine. Chronic thiamine deficiency leads to nerve cell degeneration, the scarring of the central nervous system, and atrophy of the cerebellum and peripheral nerves (1). Affected patients develop symptoms such as difficulty walking and maintaining balance, paralysis of eye muscles, confusion (Wernicke syndrome), and severe memory loss (Korsakoff syndrome). Untreated, these conditions can lead to coma and death.

Pancreatitis: Alcohol increases the risk of acute and chronic pancreatitis (1). Alcohol ingestion causes 65 percent of acute pancreatitis cases in the United States (8). Acute pancreatitis can be a life-threatening condition. Alcohol has a toxic effect on the pancreatic acinar cells that produce and store digestive enzymes. In acute pancreatitis, the digestive enzymes in the pancreas are activated while they are still in the pancreas, resulting in digestion of the pancreas and surrounding tissue. Multiple mild attacks of acute pancreatitis result in chronic pancreatitis, with extensive scarring of the pancreatic gland. The pancreatic cells, which make digestive enzymes and insulin, may be destroyed. Chronic pancreatitis patients may have diabetes, severe chronic pain, and impaired intestinal absorption of nutrients (8).

Skeletal muscle damage: Alcohol can directly damage skeletal muscle, leading to weakness and pain (1).

Reproductive system problems: Chronic alcohol use is associated with testicular atrophy (1). Decreased fertility is seen in both men and women. Pregnant women who drink alcohol have an increased risk of spontaneous abortion, and maternal alcohol use is associated with fetal damage. A single drink per day can cause the fetal alcohol syndrome associated with developmental defects, genetic malformations, and mental retardation. Fetal alcohol syndrome is the most common preventable cause of mental retardation in the United States, affecting at least 1,200 children per year (1).

OTHER SYSTEMIC EFFECTS OF CHRONIC ALCOHOL USE

- **Malnutrition:** Alcoholic beverages supply empty calories to the diet, contributing to weight gain and obesity. If alcohol is substituted for more nutrient-rich foods, malnutrition may result. Worse still, alcohol interferes with the body's metabolism of available nutrients (5). For example, alcoholics are often deficient in folate because the liver loses its ability to retain it and the kidneys increase their excretion of it (5). Low folate, the direct effects of alcohol, and the toxic effects of a breakdown product of alcohol called acetaldehyde are also associated with damage to intestinal cells and subsequent malabsorption of thiamin, folate, and vitamin B12. Liver cells damaged by alcohol have a decreased ability to activate vitamin D and vitamin A. Loss of these active nutrients can affect every cell in the body (5).

- **Cancer:** Acetaldehyde, a metabolic breakdown product of alcohol, is a tumor promoter (1). Ethanol also inhibits the breakdown of other chemical carcinogens, such as nitrosamines, which are found in cured meat such as bacon. Alcohol consumption is associated with an increased risk of several types of cancer, and this increased risk is not restricted to heavy drinkers. A study of 1.3 million British women found that even one drink per day increased the risk of cancers of the mouth, pharynx, esophagus, larynx, rectum, liver, and breast (7).

- **Addiction:** About 11 percent of American drinkers and 7.4 percent of the entire US adult population are alcoholics; this includes 11 percent of US men and 4 percent of US women (2). It is estimated that 17 percent of men and 8 percent of women will meet criteria for alcohol dependence at some point in their lives (9). One reason for the increased incidence of alcoholics in men is that men tend to have a different biochemical response to alcohol. When men drink, there is increased release of dopamine in the brain, leading to increased pleasure, reinforcement, and addiction. Common signs of alcoholism include: (5)

    A. **Tolerance:** More alcohol is needed to achieve the same degree of intoxication.

    B. **Withdrawal:** Symptoms such as anxiety, agitation, hypertension, or seizures occur when the person stops drinking.

    C. **Impaired control:** The person cannot stop after one or two drinks.

    D. **Disinterest:** The person neglects other activities, family, friends, or their job because of their drinking.

    E. **Time:** Much time is spent acquiring alcohol, drinking alcohol, or recovering from alcohol.

    F. **Impaired ability:** Intoxication or withdrawal symptoms interfere with other activities. The person is unable to function well in normal day-to-day life.

    G. **Problems:** Drinking continues despite the problems it causes.

Generally, three or more of these signs are required for a diagnosis of alcoholism.

PERSONAL OBSERVATIONS

At the risk of offending the two-thirds of the adult population that drinks, I recommend avoiding alcohol. While many light drinkers never suffer adverse effects from alcohol, over 10 percent of drinkers become alcoholics. As outlined in this chapter, the consequences to individuals and the population at large can be devastating. The only positive health consequence of drinking in moderation is a modest increase in serum high-density lipoproteins (HDLs). If you're drinking in order to increase your HDLs, try exercising more. It is more effective, and much safer.

    If you want to quit drinking but are experiencing difficulty, there are many good programs to help you. The National Alcohol Substance Abuse Information Center (NASAIC) has a website and a toll-free phone number (1-800-784-6776) available twenty-four hours a day to assist you in finding help in your area.

REFERENCES:

1. Kane AB, Kumar V. "Experimental and Nutritional Pathology." In *Robbins and Cotran Pathologic Basis of Disease*, 7th ed., edited by Kumar et al, 421–24. Philadelphia, PA: Elsevier Saunders, 2005.

2. Crawford JM. "Liver and Biliary Tract." In *Robbins and Cotran Pathologic Basis of Disease*, 7th ed., edited by Kumar et al, 904–07. Philadelphia, PA: Elsevier Saunders, 2005.

3. "Short-Term Effects of Alcohol," *Wikipedia*, accessed April 2008, http://en.wikipedia.org/wiki/Short-term_effects_of_alcohol.

4. Department of Transportation (US), National Highway Traffic Safety Administration (NHTSA). "Traffic Safety Facts 2005: Alcohol." Washington, DC, 2006.

5. Rolfes SR, Pinna K, Whitney E. *Understanding Normal and Clinical Nutrition*. 7th ed. Belmont, CA: Thomson Wadsworth, 2006: 240–49.

6. Clarke-Stewart A, Brentano C. *Divorce: Causes and Consequences*. New Haven, CT: Yale University Press, 2006.

7. Allen et al. "Moderate Alcohol Intake and Cancer Incidence in Women." *Journal of the National Cancer Institute* 101 (2009): 296–305.

8. Hruban RH, Wilentz RE. "The Pancreas." In *Robbins and Cotran Pathologic Basis of Disease*, 7th ed., edited by Kumar et al, 941–46. Philadelphia, PA: Elsevier Saunders, 2005.

9. Centers for Disease Control and Prevention. "CDC Fact Sheets: Excessive Alcohol Use and Risks to Men's Health." Atlanta, GA: CDC, April 9, 2013. http://www.cdc.gov/alcohol/fact-sheets/mens-health.htm.

9: OBESITY

The World Health Organization estimates that 1.4 billion adults and at least 40 million children younger than five are overweight (1). It is projected that 2.3 billion adults will be overweight by 2015 (1).

America is the fattest country of all, with 67 percent of the adult population categorized as overweight (2). The number of obese adults has doubled in the past twenty years. If the current trend continues, 100 percent of the US population will be overweight by 2040 (2). An especially disturbing development is that the percentage of overweight children has tripled in the past twenty years (3). It is estimated that obesity causes approximately 300,000 US deaths each year (4). Many think that obesity will soon surpass cigarette smoking as the number one preventable cause of premature death in our country.

Obesity (Fig. 9-1) has been recognized as a major risk factor for atherosclerosis by the American Heart Association (5). It is associated with high triglycerides, high amounts of bad cholesterol, and low amounts of good cholesterol. Too much fat is also closely associated with high blood pressure: 75 percent of all hypertension in the United States is attributed to obesity (5). Some speculate that the elevated blood pressure seen in overweight individuals may be due to insulin resistance and subsequent high insulin levels, which increase sodium retention and expand blood volume (6).

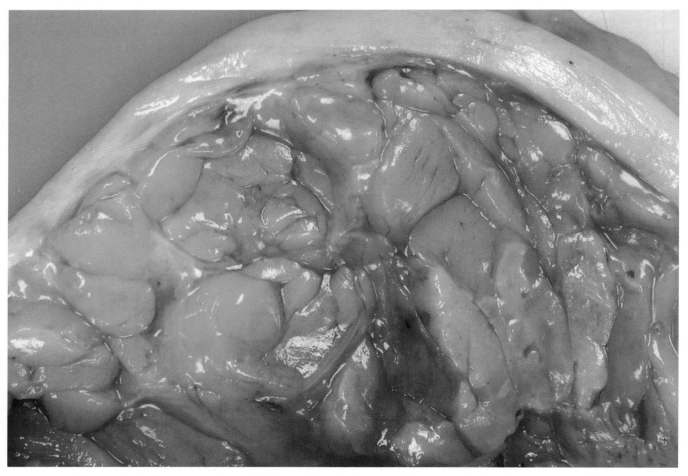

Figure 9-1: Cross section of skin and soft tissue with expanded subcutaneous fat.
The tan structure on top is skin.

Obesity may contribute to atherosclerosis in other ways that are not completely understood. As you may remember from the chapter on atherosclerosis, damage to endothelial cells, which line the inside of our arteries, is usually the first step in developing atherosclerosis. A recent study found that endothelial cell function was impaired when normal-weight individuals gained an average of nine pounds, despite no changes in blood pressure (17). The endothelial dysfunction was most closely related to gains in belly fat and returned to normal when the extra weight was lost.

Obesity causes up to 90 percent of type 2 diabetes (5). As you know from chapter 5, there are many significant problems associated with that disease. In addition, obesity is associated with an increased risk for many cancers, including breast cancer, esophageal and stomach cancers, colon cancer, endometrial cancer, and carcinomas of the kidney (5). Some hormone-dependent cancers such as endometrial cancer and breast cancer are likely stimulated by estrogens produced in fat. The reasons behind obesity's increased incidence of other cancers are uncertain (6).

Other illnesses associated with obesity include arthritis, gallstones (Fig. 9-2), carpal tunnel syndrome, chronic venous insufficiency, deep vein thrombosis with pulmonary emboli (Fig. 9-3), renal disease, gout, heat disorders, impaired immunity, impaired respiratory function, increased wound infections, female infertility, liver disease, childbirth complications, increased surgical complications, back pain, sleep apnea, pancreatitis, and urinary incontinence (5).

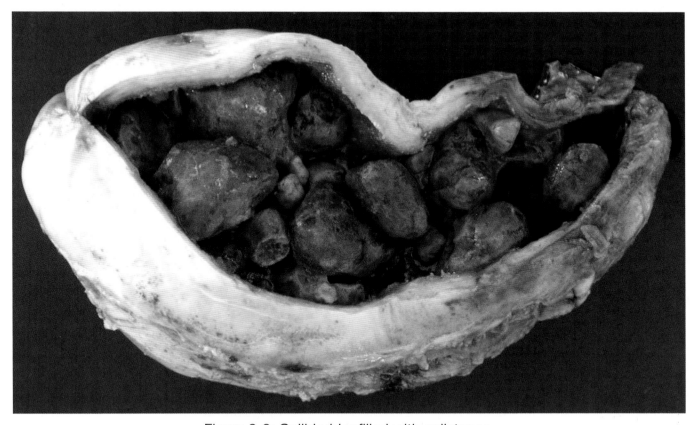

Figure 9-2: Gallbladder filled with gallstones.

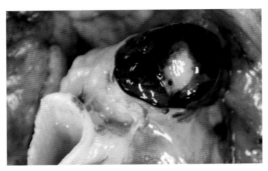

Figure 9-3: Fatal pulmonary embolus in pulmonary artery. Obese patients have an increased incidence of deep vein thrombosis (in which a clot forms within a deep vein) in the legs and pelvis. These clots can dislodge and travel through the heart to obstruct the pulmonary artery, causing sudden death.

Obesity not only causes disease, it also makes the diagnosis more difficult. Physical exams are more complicated and less informative. Radiographic studies such as X-rays, CT scans, MRIs, and ultrasounds are also hampered because of image distortion due to the excess fat. It has been estimated that fat distorts 10 to 15 percent of all images of obese patients (18). Image distortion plus fatty change (accumulation of fat in liver cells) can cause CT findings simulating liver tumors (Fig. 9-4).

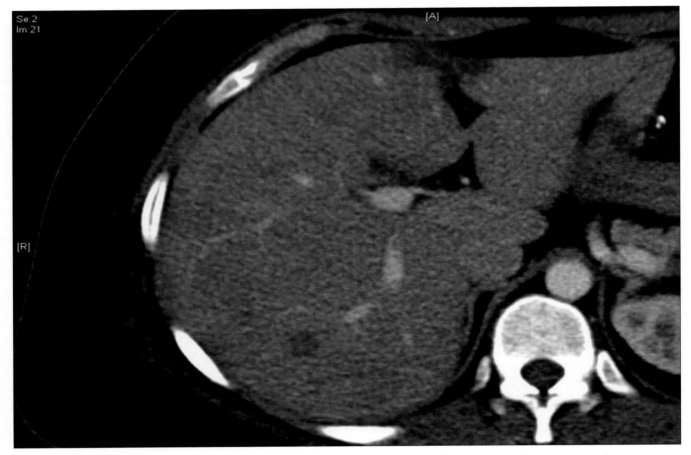

Figure 9-4: CT scan of obese patient showing dark spots in the liver resembling metastatic cancer. Biopsy showed only fatty change (see Figure 9-5). Photo courtesy of Don Howard, MD.

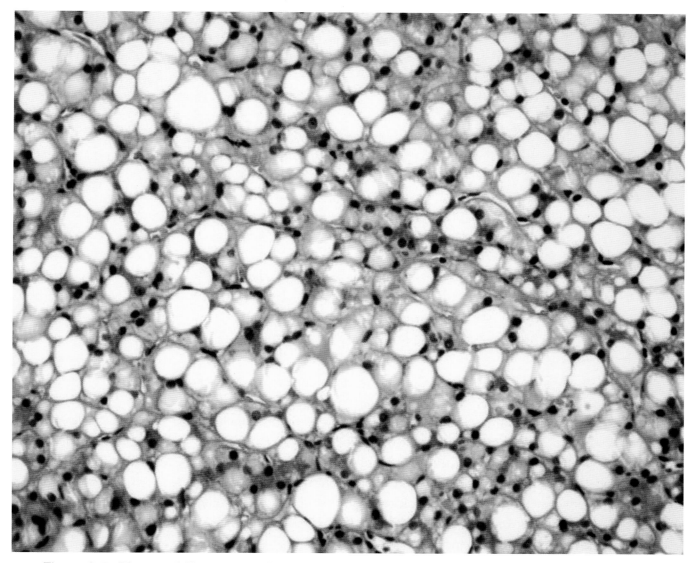

Figure 9-5: Biopsy of "liver mass" illustrated in Figure 9-4, showing only marked fatty change.

Morbidly obese patients may find that some radiographic studies cannot be performed on them at all. Many CT or MRI scanners have a table capacity limit of 350 pounds.

DEFINING AND MEASURING OBESITY

Many methods are available to assess body fat (7):

1. **Fat-fold measurements:** Body fat is estimated using calipers to measure skin-fold thicknesses at various body sites, such as the back of the upper arm, abdomen, and mid-thigh. The measurements are then compared with tables that correlate fat-fold thicknesses with percentage of body fat.

2. **Hydrodensitometry:** The patient is measured on land and again once they are submerged in water. Using the difference of the two weights, the body's volume is calculated. Using body volume, body weight, and a mathematical equation published in 1961, the doctor can estimate the patient's percentage of body fat.

3. **Bioelectrical impedance:** A low-intensity electrical current is passed through the body. Lean body tissues have less resistance to currents than fat. By measuring electrical resistance and using a mathematical formula published in 1988, the doctor can estimate the percentage of body fat.

4. **Air displacement plethysmography:** A person sits in a chamber as computerized sensors measure the air displaced by the body. Body composition is then calculated.
5. **Dual-energy X-ray absorptiometry (DXA):** Low-dose X-rays are used to differentiate fat from lean tissue in order to measure a patient's body fat.
6. **Body mass index (BMI):** The BMI uses the formula below to describe relative weight for height:

BMI = weight (lbs) multiplied by 703 divided by height (inches) squared
In metric measurements, BMI = weight (kg) divided by height (meters) squared

Example:
To calculate the BMI of a 6-foot (72-inch) man who weighs 170 pounds:
BMI = 170 x 703 divided by (72 x 72) = 23

BMI is interpreted as follows (7):
BMI < 18.5 = underweight
BMI 18.5 to 24.9 = healthy weight
BMI 25 to 29.9 = overweight
BMI > 30 = obese
BMI > 40 = extremely obese

Of the methods of measuring body fat described here, hydrodensitometry and the DXA scan are considered the most accurate. However, their use is limited due to their expense and complexity.

Because it is cheaper and easier than other measurements of body fat, BMI is the most commonly used method to determine obesity. While it usually corresponds well to other methods of estimating body fat, BMI only reflects weight for a given height; it does not directly measure body composition. As a result, muscular individuals with low body fat may be erroneously classified as overweight or even obese. For example, at the peak of his bodybuilding career, Arnold Schwarzenegger won the Mr. Olympia competition with a BMI of 31 (7).

PREVENTION/TREATMENT

The combination of a sedentary modern lifestyle and a shift to more energy-dense, processed foods has been a major factor contributing to obesity today. Marketdata Enterprises, a research firm that follows niche markets, estimates that Americans spend $60 billion a year trying to lose weight. Despite all of the effort and money spent on this problem, the incidence of obesity continues to soar. Truthfully, the formula for weight loss is simple: To lose weight, you have to burn more calories than you take in. (Notice I didn't say it was easy.)

The National Weight Control Registry, established in 1994, is tracking over 10,000 individuals who have lost significant amounts of weight and kept it off. They have a database of people who have lost thirty pounds or more and have kept it off for at least one year. How did they do it? Eighty-nine percent changed their diets and increased physical activity. Eighty-eight percent limited some type of food, especially those containing high fat and calorie counts. Ninety-two percent exercised at home; walking was the most common activity reported.

RECOMMENDATIONS FOR ENCOURAGING WEIGHT LOSS

1. **Make permanent lifestyle changes that will contribute positively to your health.** Many fad diets can result in quick weight loss but are too unhealthy or too unpleasant for a permanent lifestyle change. The result is rapid weight gain when the person goes back to his or her old way of life. Successful changes will be sustainable and contribute to your health over the long haul. Examples of such changes would be exercising more and eating healthier, less fattening foods. Such changes require some adjustments. But eventually, many find that they actually prefer their new diets and look forward to their workouts. The key to success often is in making changes that you can maintain long enough to make a habit. If you decide to join a high-impact aerobics class across town that adds two hours to your daily routine and costs $200 a month, you will likely be tempted to quit. If you can find a way to seamlessly add exercise to your daily routine, such as walking or biking to work or the local store, you may find it easier to stick with it.

2. **Understand energy balance.** The kilocalorie (kcal), commonly referred to simply as a calorie, is a unit of heat energy used to measure energy balance. When intake of energy (food) equals the output of energy (calories burned), weight remains stable. When intake exceeds output (resulting in positive energy balance), weight gain occurs. When input is less than output (resulting in negative energy balance), weight loss occurs. A pound of fat contains 3,500 kcal. A negative energy balance of 500 kcal per day will result in a loss of one pound of fat per week. The caloric content of different food components vary. Protein, for example, has 4 kcal per gram, as do carbohydrates. Fat has 9 kcal per gram and alcohol has 7 kcal per gram (7). Energy output of different activities varies with the intensity and duration of the activity and the weight of the person.

TABLE 9A
CALORIES BURNED BY VARIOUS ACTIVITIES (7)

ACTIVITY	CAL/LB/MINUTE	CAL/MINUTE IN 150 LB PERSON
Walking (3.5 mph)	.035	5.2
Running (7.5 mph)	.094	14.1
Swimming (45 yd/min)	.058	8.7
Basketball (full court)	.097	14.6
Weight lifting (vigorous)	.048	7.2
Aerobic dance (vigorous)	.062	9.3
Soccer (vigorous)	.097	14.6
Wheelchair basketball	.084	12.6
Golf (carrying clubs)	.045	6.8

Formula:

Calories burned = weight x duration of activity in minutes x cal/lb/minute

Example:

A 150-lb man who plays vigorous soccer for sixty minutes would burn 150 x 60 x .097 = 873 calories

1. **Don't eat unless you are really hungry.** It is easy to eat for other reasons, especially when you are stimulated by the sight of food, or if you are bored, thirsty, or depressed. For some people, certain times of day, or events such as celebrations, can be particularly difficult in terms of controlling your appetite. Evidence for this behavior can be seen by blood levels of leptin in obesity. Leptin is a hormone

produced in fat tissue in proportion to the amount of body fat. It works to inhibit appetite. Obese individuals tend to overeat despite high leptin levels (8).

2. **Stop eating before you are full.** When you eat, a variety of hormones such as peptide YY, pancreatic polypeptide, glucagon-like peptide 1, oxyntomodulin, amylin, and cholecystokinin are released from the gastrointestinal tract in response to the stretching of the stomach and different nutrients in food (8). These hormones travel to the brain to tell you that you are full. The problem is, it usually takes about thirty minutes for these hormones to reach their peak (8). This explains why you often feel more full thirty minutes after a meal than when you first stopped eating. A recent study found that eating quickly until full tripled the risk of obesity (9). Make a deal with yourself: Stop eating before you are full but allow yourself to eat more if you are really hungry an hour later. You will save calories in the long run.

3. **Eat low-calorie, high-volume foods.** Portion size directly correlates with a food's satiety—in other words, how well the food suppresses hunger (7). Choosing low-calorie, bulky foods such as fresh fruits and vegetables allows one to fill up on fewer calories. An added benefit is that these foods are usually more nutritious than fatty, energy-dense foods. Example: A large order of French fries contains over 500 calories. A half cup serving of green beans has about 20 calories. If you choose the green beans, you could eat ten servings (five cups!) and still save 300 calories over the one order of French fries.

4. **Eat more fiber than fat.** This is another way to guide you toward filling, nutritious, low-calorie foods. By eating more grams of fiber than fat during most meals, you will likely find that you are satisfied with fewer calories and a healthier diet. Concentrate on vegetables, fruits, grains, soy products, and nonfat dairy products such as skim milk, yogurt, and frozen yogurt. Be careful not to completely eliminate fats. Omega-3 and omega-6 fatty acids are essential for health and can be found in vegetable oils, seeds, nuts, and fish. Most people on a typical Western diet consume plenty of omega-6 fatty acids but may not get enough omega-3 fatty acids. Regular consumption of omega-3 fatty acids helps protect your heart by decreasing blood clots, preventing irregular heartbeats, and lowering blood pressure. Good sources of omega-3 fatty acids include salmon, herring, mackerel, sardines, walnuts, flaxseed oil, canola oil, and soybean oil. Replacing saturated and trans fats with monounsaturated fats and polyunsaturated fats can lower cholesterol and help prevent heart disease. This can be accomplished by avoiding foods like fatty meats, baked goods with trans fats, and high-fat dairy products, and eating more avocados, olive oil, nuts, and seeds. If you are not used to a high-fiber diet, you may experience increased intestinal gas if you dramatically increase your fiber intake. Don't worry, it will pass. (Sorry, couldn't help myself!) These symptoms can be minimized by gradually increasing your fiber intake. An example of this principle is choosing two apples for dessert (140 calories, 6 grams of fiber, 0 grams of fat) rather than a piece of apple pie (411 calories, 2 grams of fiber, 19 grams of fat). While this type of dietary change may be difficult at first, you will gradually lose your cravings for high-calorie foods laden with fat and sugar. If you still want something sweet after a fruit dessert, try eating a small piece of your favorite candy. You will still save many calories in the long run.

5. **Drink water.** The average US adult ingests about 300 calories of sugary beverages per day including soda, sports drinks, and fruit drinks (10). Moderate consumption of alcoholic beverages can easily add an additional few hundred calories. Water is cheap, healthy, and calorie free. Saving 300+ calories a day by drinking water could translate into a weight loss of thirty pounds per year. Sometimes we eat when our bodies need water more than calories. By drinking water before and during a meal we may become satisfied with fewer calories. Drinking a couple of glasses of water after a high-fiber meal can also help fill your stomach and satisfy your hunger.

6. **Swap your condiments.** Condiments can contribute greatly to your caloric intake. A baked potato with its skin included is a healthy food, with 220 calories, 4 grams of fiber, and less than 1 gram of fat. You can smother it with 10 tablespoons of salsa and add only 20 to 50 calories (7). Use the same amount of butter and you'll add 1,080 calories and 120 grams of fat (7)! Still like the taste of butter?

Try fat-free Butter Buds or butter spray to satisfy your craving with only a fraction of the calories. Spices such as garlic, mustard, vinegar, hot pepper sauce, and tomato-based sauces are usually low-calorie ways to flavor foods. Condiments featuring bases of cream or cheese, and fatty salad dressings, can add a load of calories. If you have the craving for ranch dressing (146 calories per two tablespoons), mayonnaise (about 200 calories per two tablespoons) or tartar sauce (144 calories per two tablespoons), look for low-fat versions, which may have less than half the calories. Another method to cut calories is to dilute these condiments with nonfat plain yogurt or cottage cheese. You'll get similar flavor and consistency with less fat and higher nutrition.

7. **Change your cooking methods.** The caloric content of food can easily double if it is breaded or deep fried in fats or oils. Choose other cooking methods such as broiling, baking, or grilling to save calories.

8. **Exercise.** Increasing energy output through exercise makes it much easier to lose weight. Many people know avid exercisers who eat like a horse and yet manage to stay thin. How is this possible? Because exercise does all of the following:

   A. **BURNS CALORIES.** You don't have to run marathons to lose weight from exercise. Any type of physical activity will burn calories. Look for a variety of activities that are simple, enjoyable, and easy to fit into your schedule. Walking is one of the best activities, but gardening or golf can also be effective. If you have joint problems, consider swimming or water aerobics. Don't overexert yourself, or you risk losing interest. Have fun! Your success depends more on your ability to keep exercising rather than the intensity of your workouts.

   B. **SUPPRESSES APPETITE.** Exercise not only burns calories but it also makes hunger go away. Studies have found that aerobic exercise such as running is associated with a drop in ghrelin, a hormone that stimulates appetite, and increased levels of peptide YY, a hormone that suppresses appetite (11). Resistance exercise such as weight lifting is also associated with decreased ghrelin levels (11). In either form of vigorous activity, hunger decreases both during exercise and for a short time—up to two hours—after exercise (11).

   C. **PRESERVES MUSCLE MASS.** Up to 28 percent of the weight lost by dieters who do not exercise comes from lost muscle mass (12, 13). Since muscle consumes calories at rest, losing muscle mass decreases the number of calories your body uses and makes it easier for you to gain the weight back. Preserving muscle mass will also help make you stronger and less prone to injury. Much less muscle is lost if you include exercise in your weight-loss program (12, 13).

   D. **IMPROVES GENERAL HEALTH.** (See chapter 12.)

1. **Rule out endocrine disorders.** Most cases of obesity are simply due to the person taking in more calories than what is burned, and can be reversed with lifestyle changes. However, some endocrine disorders may also cause people to be overweight. Examples include hypothyroidism, a condition that results when your body doesn't make enough thyroid hormones, and hypercortisolism (Cushing's syndrome), a condition that results when the adrenal glands make too much cortisol. Endocrine disorders should especially be considered if you notice weight gain without experiencing a change in lifestyle, if you have other symptoms, or if you do not respond to lifestyle changes that previously resulted in weight loss. Other symptoms associated with hypothyroidism include fatigue, apathy, mental sluggishness, intolerance to cold temperatures, shortness of breath, constipation, and decreased sweating (14). Other signs and symptoms of Cushing's syndrome include a round, moon-like face; the accumulation of fat in the trunk, posterior, neck, and back; weakness; fatigue; increased body hair; diabetes; lost muscle mass with weakness; easy bruising; poor wound healing; scar-like stripes on the skin, particularly on the sides of the abdomen; mental changes; osteoporosis; and menstrual abnormalities (14). Treatment of either disease can prevent serious consequences. See a doctor if you suspect that you may have an endocrine disorder.

2. **Get enough sleep.** Sleep deprivation can alter blood levels of hormones that regulate appetite, resulting in increased hunger (16).

3. **Chew your food thoroughly.** Studies have shown that chewing your food thirty to forty times results in hormonal changes that make you feel full and reduce food intake. Specifically, blood levels of glucagon-like peptide 1, peptide YY, and cholecystokinin are increased while blood levels of ghrelin are decreased. I have noticed that my hunger sometimes decreases the instant food is in my mouth. This could be explained by these hormonal changes brought on by chewing. I've experimented to see if chewing gum could help stave off hunger, and it seems to work for me. You may want to give it a try.

4. **Don't overdo it.** While the general population is getting fatter, our society's ideals for body weight are getting thinner and thinner, particularly for women. For the past forty years, most women winning Miss America, our nation's icon of beauty, have had a BMI of less than 18.5, a level considered underweight and associated with health problems (7). While some small-framed, avid exercisers may be a healthy weight even with a BMI this low, self-starvation for the sake of fashion or beauty is dangerous. Eating too little food can cause nutritional deficiencies, osteoporosis, amenorrhea (a loss of menstrual periods), lethargy, depression, and poor immunity with increased infections. It is ironic that while the incidence of obesity in the general population is increasing, the incidence of anorexia nervosa is increasing in girls and young women. Anorexia nervosa is a condition associated with dangerously low food intake, very low body weight, distorted body image (the person thinks they are plump even when they are very underweight), and an irrational fear of being overweight. This disorder eventually kills between 5 and 20 percent of those affected, making it the most deadly mental illness. While all parts of the body are affected, the bones and heart show the most damage. Bones become weak and break easily. The heart loses so much muscle mass that it can fail, causing death. You don't have to have the full anorexia syndrome for undereating to harm your health. Underweight individuals regardless of cause show an increased death rate compared to those of a normal weight (15). An ideal goal? To make health and fitness your ultimate priority rather than trying to achieve a certain appearance.

PERSONAL OBSERVATIONS

I've seen pathology specimens from many diseases caused by obesity including cancer, gangrene, heart attacks, hepatitis, and arthritis. Obesity is challenging smoking as the number one cause of preventable death. In fact, many experts now consider obesity to be the most important health problem in America. The rapid rise of obesity has come about because of the overall reduction in exercise and increased consumption of high-calorie foods. Fortunately, lifestyle changes are very effective in weight control. By making the simple changes outlined in this chapter, you can achieve and maintain your optimal weight. Focus on making changes in your routine that you can keep long-term. Many find it beneficial to enlist the help and support of friends and family. You can also find support through free online resources such as www.sparkpeople.com and www.weightlossbuddy.com.

REFERENCES:

1. World Health Organization. "Obesity and Overweight: Fact Sheet 311." March 2013. http://www.who.int/mediacentre/factsheets/fs311/en/.

2. Heaner M. "Obesity in America." http://health.msn.com/reports/obesity/articlepage.aspx?cp-documentid=100168553.

3. Centers for Disease Control and Prevention. "Prevalence of Overweight among Children and Adolescents: United States, 2003–2004." Atlanta, GA: CDC, April 6, 2010. http://www.cdc.gov/nchs/data/hestat/overweight/overweight_child_03.htm.

4. Satcher D. "The Surgeon General's Call to Action to Prevent and Decrease Overweight and Obesity 2001." US Department of Health and Human Services. Washington, DC: HHS, 2000.

5. American Obesity Association. "Health Effects of Obesity: AOA Fact Sheets." May 2005.

6. Kane AB, Kumar V. "Environmental and Nutritional Pathology." In *Robbins and Cotran Pathologic Basis of Disease*, 7th ed., edited by Kumar et al, 461–65. Philadelphia, PA: Elsevier Saunders, 2005.

7. Rolfes SR, Pinna K, Whitney E. *Understanding Normal and Clinical Nutrition*. 7th ed. Belmont, CA: Thomson Wadsworth, 2006: 250–318, H1-83.

8. Neary MT, Batterham RL. "Gut Hormones: Implications for the Treatment of Obesity." *Pharmacology & Therapeutics* 124 (2009): 44–56.

9. Maruyama et al. "The Joint Impact on Being Overweight of Self-Reported Behaviours of Eating Quickly and Eating until Full: Cross Sectional Survey." *British Medical Journal* 337 (2008): a2002.

10. Bleich et al. "Increasing Consumption of Sugar-Sweetened Beverages among US Adults: 1988-1994 to 1999-2004." *American Journal of Clinical Nutrition* 89 (2009): 372–81.

11. Broom et al. "Influence of Resistance and Aerobic Exercise on Hunger, Circulating Levels of Acylated Ghrelin, and Peptide YY in Healthy Males." *American Journal of Physiology—Regulatory, Integrative and Comparative Physiology* 296 (2009): R29–R35.

12. Ballor DL, Poehlman ET. "Exercise-Training Enhances Fat-Free Mass Preservation during Diet-Induced Weight Loss: A Meta-Analytical Finding." *International Journal of Obesity and Related Metabolic Disorders* 18, no. 1 (January 1994): 35–40.

13. Wood et al. "Changes in Plasma Lipids and Lipoproteins in Overweight Men during Weight Loss through Dieting as Compared with Exercise." *New England Journal of Medicine* 319 (1988): 1173–79.

14. Maitra A, Abbas AK. "The Endocrine System." In *Robbins and Cotran Pathologic Basis of Disease*, 7th ed., edited by Kumar et al, 1155–1226. Philadelphia, PA: Elsevier Saunders, 2005.

15. Flegal et al. "Excess Deaths Associated with Underweight, Overweight, and Obesity." *Journal of the American Medical Association* 293 (2005): 1861–67.

16. Spiegel et al. "Sleep Curtailment in Healthy Young Men Is Associated with Decreased Leptin Levels, Elevated Ghrelin Levels, and Increased Hunger and Appetite." *Annals of Internal Medicine* 141, no. 11 (December 7, 2004): 846–50.

17. Romero-Corral et al. "Modest Visceral Fat Gain Causes Endothelial Dysfunction in Healthy Humans." *Journal of the American College of Cardiology* 56 (2010): 662–66.

18. Radiological Society of North America. "Patient Size a Weighty Problem for Radiologists." December 2005. http://www.rsna.org/uploadedfiles/rsna/content/news/dec2005.pdf.

10: SEXUALLY TRANSMITTED DISEASES

The World Health Organization estimates that 340 million new cases of curable sexually transmitted diseases, such as syphilis, gonorrhea, and chlamydia, occur each year (1). Worldwide, AIDS is the leading cause of death in women between the ages of fifteen and forty-four (2). Up to 80 percent of the population is exposed to human papillomavirus, the virus involved with the development of most genital cancers, during their lifetime (3, 6). In the United States, 26 percent of girls between the ages of fourteen and nineteen already have at least one sexually transmitted disease (4). These diseases cause millions of deaths and much suffering each year. And almost all could be prevented.

A mutually faithful monogamous sexual relationship with someone who has had no other partners virtually eliminates the risk of sexually transmitted disease.

The most common sexually transmitted diseases are discussed in this chapter.

HUMAN PAPILLOMAVIRUS (HPV)

Human papillomavirus is a group of over 100 related viruses (5). HPV is the most common sexually transmitted infection in the United States. About 20 million Americans are currently infected, and 6.2 million US citizens get a new HPV infection each year (6). It is estimated that 80 percent of women are infected with HPV by the time they are fifty years of age (6). More than thirty types of HPV can be transmitted through sexual contact (5). Because HPV does not usually cause symptoms, people often do not know they have it, nor are they conscious of infecting their partners (6).

The infection becomes evident when tumors begin to form. Some types of HPV, such as HPV types 6 and 11, are associated with genital warts known as condyloma acuminatum (Fig. 10-1). These types are referred to as "low risk" HPV since they are rarely associated with cancer. Other HPV types, such as types 16, 18, 31, 33, 35, 39, 45, 51, 52, 56, 58, 59, 66, 68, and 73, are known as "high risk" HPV since they are frequently associated with cancers of the uterine cervix, vulva, and penis (5). Most of these HPV-induced cancers are squamous cell carcinomas (Fig.10-2). However, adenocarcinomas of the cervix can also be caused by these viruses (Fig. 10-3).

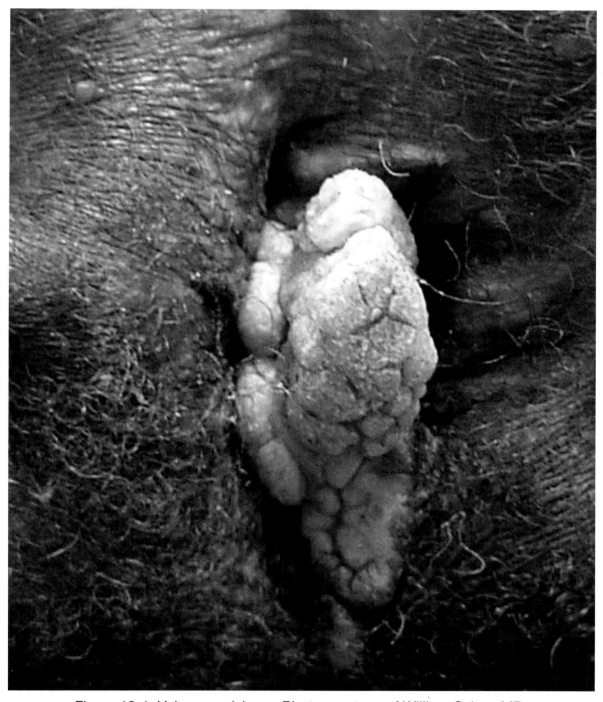

Figure 10-1: Vulvar condyloma. Photo courtesy of William Salzer, MD.

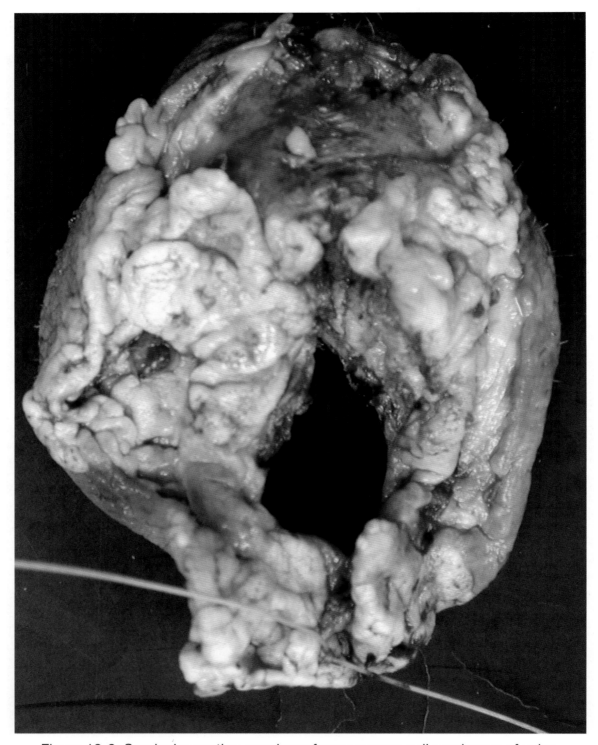

Figure 10-2: Surgical resection specimen for squamous cell carcinoma of vulva.

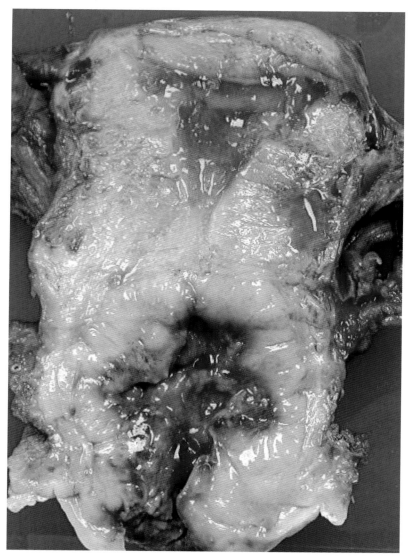

Figure 10-3: Adenocarcinoma of cervix.

Most HPV-induced cancers arise from precancerous mucosal proliferations called dysplasia. Squamous dysplasia may exist for years before invasive cancer develops. This gives patients and doctors a window of opportunity to cure HPV-related cellular proliferations before a cancer even develops. The Pap smear has been very effective in detecting dysplastic lesions of the uterine cervix, decreasing the death rate due to cervical cancer. Sixty years ago, cervical cancer was the leading cause of cancer death in US women (3). Because of Pap smears, the death rate from this disease has subsequently declined by two-thirds (3). However, despite these advances, each year in the US about 11,000 women are diagnosed with cervical cancer, 3,400 women are diagnosed with vulvar cancer, 2,200 women are diagnosed with vaginal cancer, 1,200 men are diagnosed with penile cancer, and 5,000 people (3,000 women and 2,000 men) are diagnosed with anal cancer (7). The incidence of cervical cancer is much higher in cultures where Pap smears are not routinely performed, while the incidence of penile cancers is ten to twenty times higher in cultures where circumcision is not routinely practiced. It is thought that circumcision is associated with a lower incidence of infection by HPV. Circumcision also helps prevent the buildup of debris called smegma, which may contain carcinogens that work with HPV infections to cause cancer (8).

PREVENTION/TREATMENT

Condoms may lower the risk of developing some HPV-related diseases, such as genital warts and cervical cancer, but they do not fully protect against HPV, since HPV can infect areas not covered by a condom. A recently developed HPV vaccine called Gardasil protects against HPV subtypes 6, 11, 16, and 18, which together cause 70 percent of cervical cancers and 90 percent of genital warts (9). There is no effective treatment for HPV (9). The virus may go away on its own. If it doesn't, treatment is directed against the dysplasias and tumors it causes.

Early detection and treatment of these lesions would prevent almost all cancer deaths. Ladies, get your annual Pap smears. Anyone with growths in the genital or anal region should see their doctor without delay.

ACQUIRED IMMUNODEFICIENCY SYNDROME (AIDS)

AIDS is a disease caused by the human immunodeficiency virus (HIV). While it is a relatively new disease, with the first cases being reported in 1981, it has been a modern plague, killing more than 25 million people (10). Over 33 million people, including 2.5 million children, are living with HIV. Each year about 2.5 million people become newly infected with HIV, and over 2 million people die of AIDS (10). In the United States, AIDS is the second leading cause of death in men between the ages of twenty-five and forty-four, and the third leading cause of death for women in this age group (11).

Over 75 percent of HIV cases are spread through sexual contact. Most of the remaining cases are acquired through intravenous drug use or transmitted from a mother to her baby (11). A very small percentage of cases are transmitted through blood transfusions or acquired through accidents, such as needlesticks in health care settings. HIV infection occurs when there is a transfer of blood or bodily fluids containing the virus. Sexual transmission occurs through the transfer of the virus in semen, vaginal secretions, or blood. The risk of acquiring HIV is increased when there are other coexisting sexually transmitted diseases, such as syphilis, herpes, gonorrhea, and chlamydia (11). Transmission among intravenous drug abusers occurs by sharing needles or syringes with contaminated blood. Mother-to-infant transmission occurs through the placenta, during delivery through an infected birth canal, and after birth by ingestion of contaminated breast milk.

Once HIV enters the body, it infects cells of the immune system responsible for fighting infections. HIV particularly targets cells called helper T cells, the master regulators of immunity that control other cells that fight infections. In an active infection, approximately 100 billion new viral particles are produced, and 1 to 2 billion helper T cells die each day (11). By eliminating helper T cells, HIV effectively destroys the immune system (11).

The natural history of HIV infection has three phases (11):

1. **Acute viral syndrome:** This phase develops three to six weeks after infection and generally resolves in two to four weeks. It is characterized by a flu-like illness with sore throat, muscle aches, fever, weight loss, and fatigue. Enlarged lymph nodes, diarrhea, vomiting, or a rash may also occur.

2. **Chronic phase:** This phase is marked by the continued proliferation of the virus, but relative control of it by the immune system. It may last for years. Patients in this phase may have minor infections such as thrush (a fungal infection in the mouth) or shingles. Patients may not feel sick during this phase. It is probable that most cases of HIV infection are spread from patient to partner in the chronic phase.

3. **Acquired immunodeficiency syndrome (AIDS):** In this phase, the HIV overwhelms the immune system. With the immune system disabled, patients develop serious infections and cancers (Fig. 10-4), which ultimately lead to death.

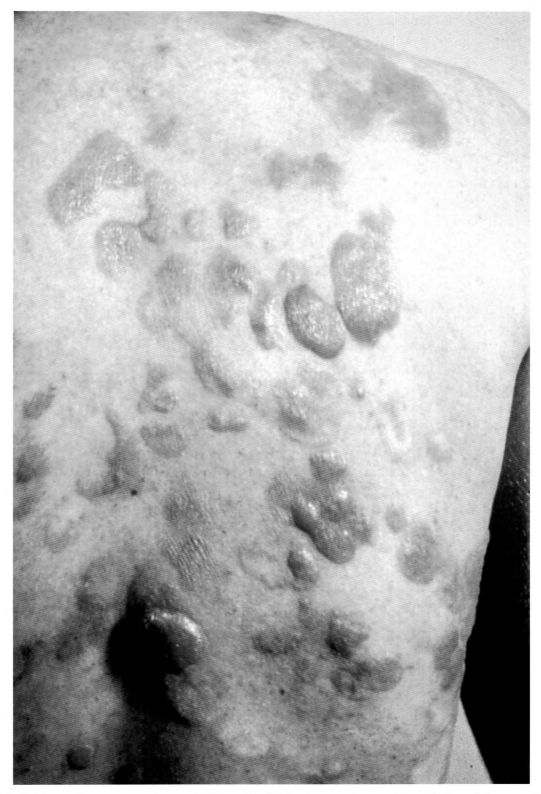

Figure 10-4: Kaposi's sarcoma in an AIDS patient. Photo courtesy of the National Cancer Institute.

PREVENTION/TREATMENT

Because HIV infection is spread mainly through sex and IV drug abuse, the epidemic could be virtually eliminated through changes in behavior. Since HIV is transmitted through blood and bodily fluids, the use of condoms can decrease sexual transmission. Thus far, efforts to develop a vaccine have been unsuccessful, though recently developed antiretroviral drugs help prevent the HIV virus from multiplying within the infected person. They have been effective in delaying the progression of HIV infection to AIDS.

CHLAMYDIA

Chlamydia trachomatis is a small bacterium that lives as an intercellular parasite. Genital infection by chlamydia is the most common bacterial sexually transmitted disease in the world (12). More than 1 million US cases were reported to the Centers for Disease Control (CDC) in 2006 (13). Chlamydia is known as a "silent" disease because about 75 percent of infected women and half of infected men have no symptoms (13). Infected individuals often unknowingly pass the disease to others.

Untreated chlamydial infection can lead to serious complications. In women, the infection can spread to the uterus or fallopian tubes, causing pelvic inflammatory disease (PID). The resulting scarring can lead to infertility, chronic pelvic pain, and ectopic pregnancies. Pelvic inflammatory disease occurs in up to 40 percent of women with untreated chlamydia (13). Infection with chlamydia also makes women up to five times more likely to be infected with HIV if exposed (13). This is because the inflammation associated with chlamydia infection brings inflammatory cells, including helper T cells, near the surface of the mucosa where they can be exposed to the HIV virus.

In men, complications are unusual; however, untreated chlamydia infection can cause epididymitis, which is the inflammation of the organ adjacent to the testis responsible for storing sperm. This condition can cause pain and sterility (13).

Infection with certain subtypes of chlamydia trachomatis causes lymphogranuloma venereum, a chronic ulcerative disease associated with swollen, tender lymph nodes and fibrotic strictures of the genital tract and anus (12).

In pregnant women, chlamydial infections can lead to premature delivery. Babies can contract the disease during birth and develop eye infections and pneumonia as a result (13).

PREVENTION/TREATMENT

Chlamydial infections can be cured with antibiotics; azithromycin or doxycycline are often used. Infected individuals should seek treatment before permanent damage occurs. Since chlamydia infections are often asymptomatic, the CDC recommends yearly chlamydia testing in sexually active women ages twenty-five and younger, older women who have a new sex partner or multiple partners, and all pregnant women (13).

GONORRHEA

Gonorrhea is caused by bacteria called Neisseria gonorrhoeae. It is estimated that more than 700,000 US citizens get new gonorrheal infections each year (14). Gonorrhea is spread through contact with the penis, vagina, mouth, or anus (14). Like chlamydia, gonorrhea is often asymptomatic, and the disease can be unknowingly passed on to others (14).

In men, gonorrhea sometimes causes urethritis, or an inflammation of the urethra, which leads to burning with urination and discharge from the penis. Some men experience painful or swollen testicles. Untreated infection can lead to epididymitis and sterility (14).

Most women have no symptoms of infection. However, untreated infection can lead to pelvic inflammatory disease (PID), causing infertility or a pregnancy outside the uterus, known as ectopic pregnancy. Ectopic pregnancies can rupture, causing serious bleeding, which may kill the mother. PID can be difficult to treat, and may be associated with chronic, severe pain (14).

Both men and women can develop a life-threatening gonorrheal blood infection known as sepsis. Once in the blood, the bacteria can infect joints. This condition is known as septic arthritis (12, 14). As with chlamydia, genital gonorrheal infections predispose patients to transmission of the human immunodeficiency virus (HIV) (14). A pregnant woman with gonorrhea may transmit the infection to her baby during delivery. This can cause the baby to develop blindness, arthritis, or sepsis (14).

PREVENTION/TREATMENT

Antibiotic therapy can cure gonorrhea. However, drug-resistant strains are developing in many areas of the world, including the United States. Condoms can reduce the risk of gonorrhea, but it is controversial how effective they are (14). Different studies have shown that condoms decrease the spread of gonorrhea from 50 percent to over 90 percent, but a problem with studies of condom use and disease is that many people don't use them consistently. Because the gonorrheal eye infections in newborns can be prevented by the application of eye drops containing silver nitrate or antibiotics, many states require them to be routinely administered after birth.

GENITAL HERPES

At least 45 million Americans ages twelve and older have a genital herpes infection (15). The disease is usually caused by herpes simplex type 2 (HSV-2). It may also be caused by herpes simplex type 1 (HSV-1), the same virus that causes fever blisters or cold sores in the mouth (12).

The disease is transmitted to women easier than men. About one in four women and one in eight men have HSV-2 in the United States (15). Clinical symptoms are only seen in about one-third of infected individuals (3), and the disease can be transmitted from patient to partner without symptoms (15). In symptomatic cases, the involved area of the genital tract develops painful red papules, which progress to blisters and then ulcers (Fig. 10-5). The blisters and ulcers contain numerous virus particles, and sexual contact with one of these lesions during active infection readily leads to transmission of the disease (3). The lesions heal in a few weeks, but the herpes virus remains present in the cells of adjacent nerves (3). About two-thirds of infected patients develop recurrent outbreaks of the lesions, and the virus remains in the body for life (3). However, the frequency of symptomatic outbreaks tends to decrease over time (15).

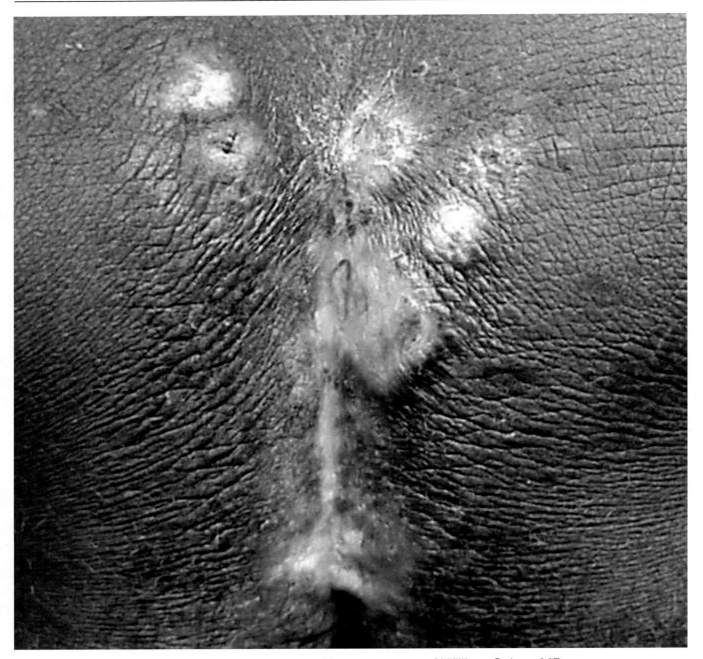

Figure 10-5: Genital herpes. Photo courtesy of William Salzer, MD.

Like many other sexually transmitted diseases, herpes can facilitate the spread of the HIV virus (15). Transmission of genital herpes from a pregnant woman to her baby during delivery can result in serious—potentially fatal—infections in the baby. Pregnant women with active genital herpes at the time of delivery may undergo cesarean section to avoid this complication (15).

PREVENTION/TREATMENT

There is no cure for genital herpes. However, antiviral medications can shorten and prevent outbreaks of the genital lesions (15). Condoms may not prevent infection since transmission can occur in areas not covered by the condom. Any genital-to-genital or oral-to-genital contact can spread the disease; sexual intercourse is not required (15).

SYPHILIS

Syphilis is caused by a corkscrew-shaped bacterium called Treponema pallidum (12). Over 12 million cases of syphilis develop each year worldwide (1). It is very common in some parts of the world, such as Africa. For example, a 2001 study of pygmies in Cameroon found that 20 percent were infected with syphilis. Public health programs and penicillin treatments have been successful in reducing the incidence of the disease in the United States. Only 5,979 cases were reported in 2000 (12). Unfortunately, the number of US cases has recently been rebounding, and 46,000 cases were reported in 2011 (12).

Syphilis is divided into three stages (12):

1. **Primary syphilis:** This first stage occurs approximately three weeks after sexual contact with the infected individual; a firm, non-tender, raised red lesion called a chancre develops where the bacteria has invaded the exposed genital area. The chancre heals in three to six weeks with or without therapy.

2. **Secondary syphilis:** This second stage develops in approximately three-quarters of untreated patients two to ten weeks after the chancre. It is due to the spread of the bacteria within skin and mucus membranes. Patients develop a rash, most frequently on their palms or soles (Fig. 10-6). Moist areas of skin may have elevated plaques called condyloma lata. Sores on mucus membranes, enlarged lymph nodes, mild fever, malaise, and weight loss are also common. The symptoms of secondary syphilis last for several weeks, but then disappear.

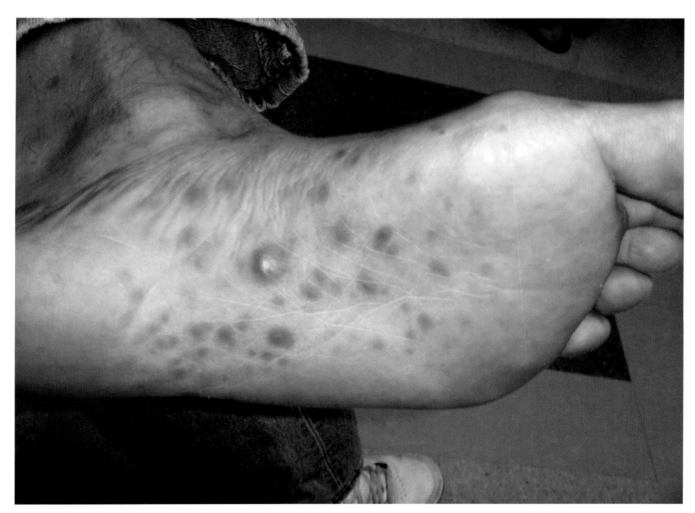

Figure 10-6: Secondary syphilis. Photo courtesy of William Salzer, MD.

3. **Tertiary syphilis:** The third stage of the disease occurs in approximately one-third of untreated patients, usually after an asymptomatic period of five years or more. Inflammation of the aorta, the main artery that distributes blood from the heart to the rest of the body, occurs in more than 80 percent of the cases. Inflammation and the narrowing of the small arteries that supply the outer portions of the aorta with blood leads to scarring and aneurysms, which are dilations of the artery. Aortic aneurysms may cause death via two mechanisms: They may rupture, resulting in a fatal hemorrhage, or the dilation of the aorta may lead to the dilation of the aortic valve in the heart. Malfunction of this valve can cause heart failure.

About 10 percent of patients with tertiary syphilis develop infection of the brain and spinal cord. This is associated with the progressive loss of mental and physical functions, accompanied by mood alterations, dementia, and impaired sensation. The body's immune reaction to the syphilis organisms may result in ball-like pockets of inflammation called gummas throughout the body. They most commonly occur in bones, skin, the mouth, and in the upper airways, and are associated with pain, swelling, and bone fractures.

Congenital syphilis occurs when the syphilis organism crosses the placenta from an infected mother to her fetus. This happens most commonly in the primary and secondary stages of the disease. Death of the infant occurs in approximately 25 percent of untreated cases. Surviving babies may experience blindness, deafness, and other birth defects.

PREVENTION/TREATMENT

Condoms can help prevent the spread of syphilis but are not totally effective since the sores caused by this disease can occur in areas not covered by a condom. Syphilis can be diagnosed with a blood test and is easy to cure with antibiotics such as penicillin in its early stages. Once syphilis has reached the tertiary stage, antibiotics will kill the bacteria, but cannot repair tissue damage that has already occurred.

PERSONAL OBSERVATIONS

Sexually transmitted diseases are epidemic in our society and cause tremendous suffering. Fortunately, this group of diseases could be virtually eliminated by lifestyle changes. Sexual abstinence before marriage, and remaining faithful during marriage, would reduce the incidence of these diseases to near zero. You may consider this recommendation to be unrealistic, but I ask you to consider it. I have never met anyone who regretted adopting this behavior.

REFERENCES:

1. World Health Organization. "Global Prevalence and Incidence of Selected Curable Sexually Transmitted Infections Overview and Estimates." Geneva: WHO, 2001.

2. World Health Organization. "Women's Health: Fact Sheet 334." Geneva: WHO, November 2009.

3. Crum CP. "The Female Genital Tract." In *Robbins and Cotran Pathologic Basis of Disease*, 7th ed., edited by Kumar et al, 1059–79. Philadelphia, PA: Elsevier Saunders, 2005.

4. Centers for Disease Control and Prevention. "Abstract D4a—Prevalence of Sexually Transmitted Infections and Bacterial Vaginosis among Female Adolescents in the United States: Data from the National Health and Nutritional Examination Survey (NHANES) 2003–2004." National STD Prevention Conference. Atlanta, GA: CDC, March 2008.

5. National Cancer Institute. "Human Papillomaviruses and Cancer: Questions and Answers." National Cancer Institute Fact Sheet. Reviewed February 14, 2008.

6. Centers for Disease Control and Prevention. "HPV Vaccine—Questions and Answers for the Public." Atlanta, GA: CDC, June 28, 2007.

7. Centers for Disease Control and Prevention. "Genital HPV." CDC Fact Sheet. Atlanta, GA: CDC, December 2007.

8. Epstein JI. "The Lower Urinary Tract and Male Genital System." In *Robbins and Cotran Pathologic Basis of Disease*, 7th ed., edited by Kumar et al, 1035–37. Philadelphia, PA: Elsevier Saunders, 2005.

9. Centers for Disease Control and Prevention. "HPV Vaccine Questions & Answers." Atlanta, GA: CDC, August 2006.

10. UNAIDS/World Health Organization. "AIDS Epidemic Update." Geneva: WHO, November 2007.

11. Abbas AK. "Diseases of Immunity." In *Robbins and Cotran Pathologic Basis of Disease*, 7th ed., edited by Kumar et al, 245–58. Philadelphia, PA: Elsevier Saunders, 2005.

12. McAdam AJ, Sharpe AH. "Infectious Diseases." In *Robbins and Cotran Pathologic Basis of Disease*, 7th ed., 343–411. Philadelphia, PA: Elsevier Saunders, 2005.

13. Centers for Disease Control and Prevention. "Chlamydia." CDC Fact Sheet. Atlanta, GA: CDC, December 2007.

14. Centers for Disease Control and Prevention. "Gonorrhea." CDC Fact Sheet. Atlanta, GA: CDC, December 2007.

15. US Department of Health and Human Services, Office on Women's Health. "Genital Herpes—Frequently Asked Questions." Washington, DC: OWH, August 10, 2009.

11: DRUG ABUSE

Drug abuse, addiction, and overdose are common and serious health problems. Over 20 million Americans, including nearly 20 percent of young adults ages eighteen to twenty-five, are current users of illicit drugs (1). About 7 million are estimated to be drug dependent, and nearly 3 million US citizens start using drugs each year (1).

Each year in the US, illicit drug use causes about 17,000 deaths (2) and is associated with over a million hospitalizations at a cost of nearly $10 billion (3). In 2003, the cost of substance abuse treatment in the United States was estimated to be $21 billion (3).

Drug abuse is also closely associated with crime. In 1998, data from thirty-five US cities showed that from 42.5 percent to 78.7 percent of all men arrested had a positive drug test (4). Nearly a third of state prison inmates were under the influence of drugs at the time of their offense, and over 30 percent of prison inmates convicted of burglary committed the robbery with the intent to use the money to buy drugs (4). A more recent study from Great Britain estimates that between 33 percent and 50 percent of all thefts are committed by drug users, and 75 percent of people addicted to heroin or crack cocaine commit crimes to fund their habits.

Countless harmful substances have been abused, and the list constantly expands. Use of many of these drugs can lead to addiction, which can overwhelm all other aspects of a person's life to the point that their only goal is to buy and use drugs. Addiction can be due to physical dependence, where the body develops a need for the drug in order to function, or from psychological factors, such as depending on the drug to deal with stress. Sometimes drug use is associated with tolerance, in which the body adapts to the presence of the drug and a higher dose is needed to obtain the desired effect. Tolerance can be especially dangerous since higher doses of drugs are usually associated with more severe and potentially fatal side effects.

Drug abuse can rob you of your health, your dignity, and your life. It truly is good advice to "Just Say No!" Details behind the most commonly abused drugs follow.

COCAINE

Cocaine is a drug extracted from the leaves of the South American coca plant (5). Cocaine (Fig. 11-1) can be snorted, injected, or smoked.

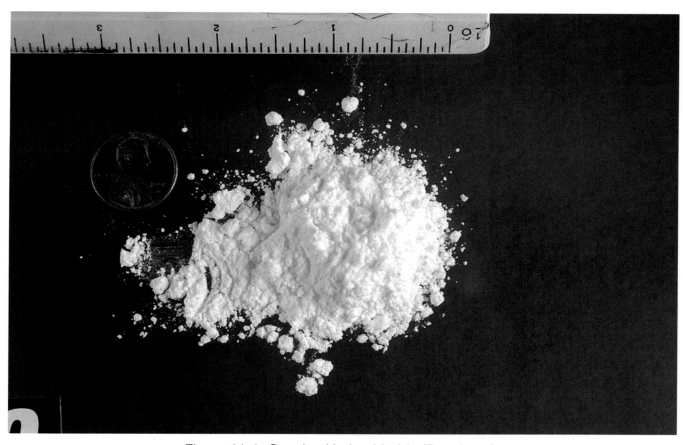

Figure 11-1: Cocaine Hydrochloride (Powdered).
Photo courtesy of the Drug Enforcement Administration.

Crack is the street name for a crystalline form of cocaine that makes a crackling sound when it is heated for smoking (Fig. 11-2).

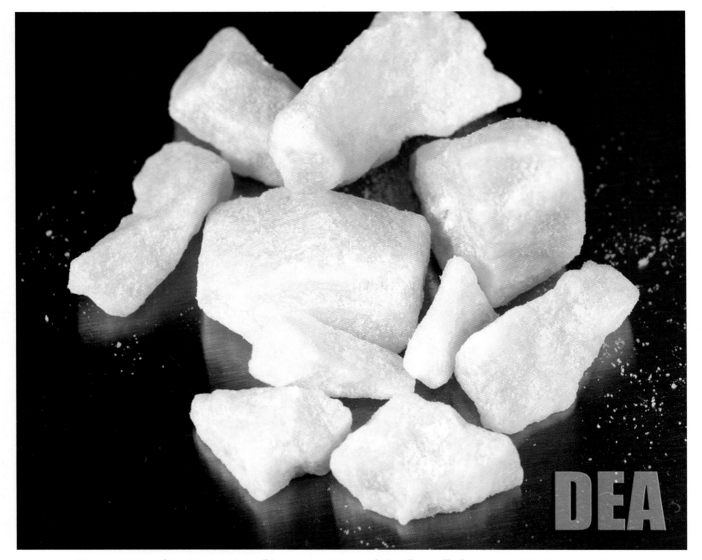

Figure 11-2: Crack cocaine. Photo courtesy of the Drug Enforcement Administration.

A 2008 survey found that 36.8 million American people, or 14.7 percent of the US population, had used cocaine at least once in their lifetime; 5.3 million, or 2.1 percent, had used it in the past year (1). About 6 percent of newborn infants will test positive for cocaine due to maternal drug abuse (5).

Cocaine blocks the reuptake of dopamine, serotonin, and catecholamines in the central nervous system. This prolongs dopamine's effects on the brain, including its pleasure centers, resulting in euphoria, paranoia, and increased energy. Unfortunately, cocaine also leads to the constriction of blood vessels throughout the body, which can cut off the blood supply to vital organs and cause serious damage (Fig. 11-3).

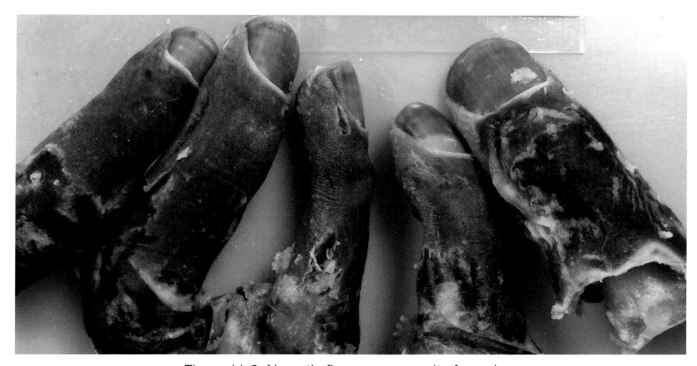

Figure 11-3: Necrotic fingers as a result of cocaine.

The constriction of vessels supplying blood to the heart can lead to death of the heart muscle; the constriction of vessels supplying blood to the brain can cause death of parts of the brain. Sudden death can result from heart attacks, cardiac arrhythmias, or stroke (5). In total, cocaine was involved in 505,224 US emergency room visits in 2011 (6).

In pregnant women, the constriction of blood vessels can result in decreased blood flow to the placenta and decreased oxygen to the fetus. Spontaneous abortion, placental abruption (when the placenta separates from the uterine wall), and hemorrhages in newborn babies can result (5).

When used with alcohol, cocaine can lead to the formation of cocaethylene in the liver. This substance intensifies cocaine's effects and is associated with a greater risk of sudden death (7).

Cocaine is highly addictive; chronic use is associated with malnutrition, loss of smell, nosebleeds, bowel gangrene, anxiety, paranoia, hallucinations, and psychosis (7). If injected, shared needles can lead to infectious diseases such as hepatitis and HIV/AIDS.

METHAMPHETAMINE

Methamphetamine is a very potent and highly addictive central nervous system stimulant. Over 12 million people in the United States have abused methamphetamine and about 1.2 million used it in 2012 (20). The drug can be taken orally, by intravenous injection, smoked, or snorted. Users use methamphetamine in powder (Fig. 11-4), rock (Fig. 11-5), or liquid form. Common street names for the drug include meth, speed, crystal meth, ice, and glass (8).

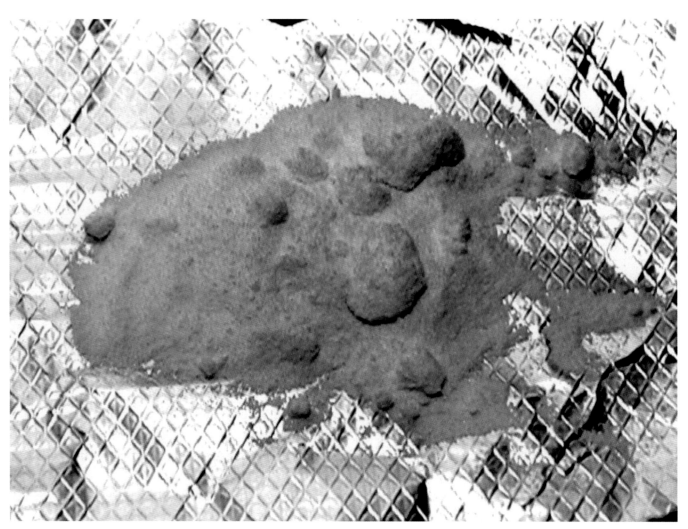

Figure 11-4: Powdered methamphetamine.
Photo courtesy of the Drug Enforcement Administration.

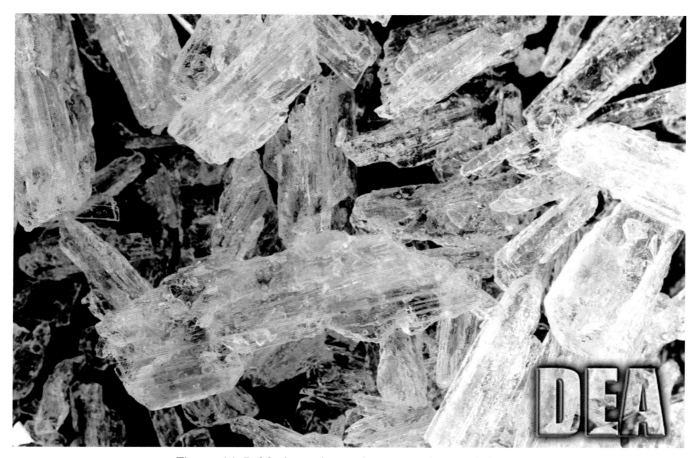

Figure 11-5: Methamphetamine, crystal or rock form.
Photo courtesy of the Drug Enforcement Administration.

In the brain, methamphetamine increases the release and blocks the reuptake of dopamine, giving users a transient rush of euphoria and energy. Other short-term effects can include elevated blood pressure, elevated body temperature, sleeplessness, irritability, paranoia, nausea, vomiting, diarrhea, headache, and uncontrollable jaw clenching; afterwards, the brain is depleted of dopamine, resulting in depression and lethargy (10). The body quickly develops a tolerance to the drug, and higher doses are required to get the desired high and to avoid the withdrawal symptoms of depression, fatigue, anxiety, and intense drug craving (8). High doses can cause delirium, seizures, irregular heartbeat, stroke, coma, and sudden death (5, 9, 10).

Methamphetamine damages brain cells containing dopamine and serotonin, two chemicals essential for normal brain function (9). Chronic abuse can cause anxiety, confusion, mood disturbances, the inability to sleep, violent behavior, paranoia, hallucinations, and delusions (such as the sensation of insects crawling under the skin) (8, 10). The fact that these mental symptoms can last years after methamphetamine abuse has ceased suggests long-lasting or even permanent brain injury (8, 9). Additional evidence of permanent brain injury can be found in recent studies that show that methamphetamine abuse increases the risk of developing Parkinson's disease.

Meth mouth is a common effect of methamphetamine abuse (11). Teeth show signs of advanced decay and degenerative changes, and they are quickly transformed into painful black stubs (Fig. 11-6).

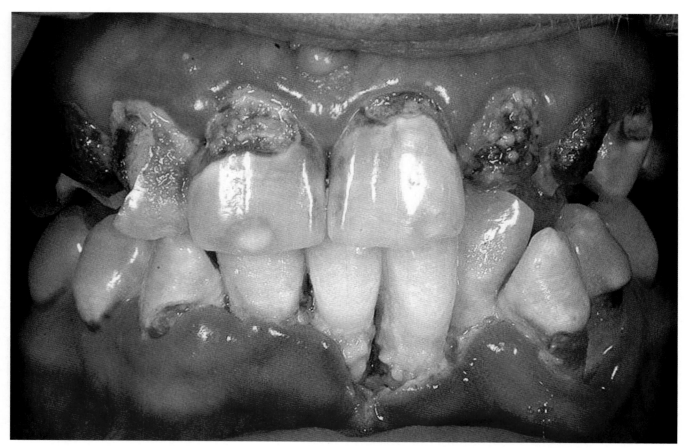

Figure 11-6: Meth mouth.
Image courtesy of Stephen Wagner, DDS, and Martin Spiller, DMD.

The causes of meth mouth are not completely understood, and several factors may contribute to its development. Methamphetamine is thought to decrease saliva production as well as the blood supply to the gums. Methamphetamine abusers also commonly experience dry mouth and crave sugary drinks such as soda. It doesn't help that addicts often neglect many basic tasks of life such as brushing their teeth. Marked jaw clenching often occurs when users experience the rush of the drug. Another potential factor for meth mouth is that methamphetamine is often contaminated by many toxic chemicals. For each pound of methamphetamine produced, six pounds of hazardous chemicals are produced in the production process. Methamphetamine bought on the street often contains many tooth-dissolving substances such as red phosphorous, lye, drain cleaner, muriatic acid, and battery acid (11, 12).

Another characteristic ailment among methamphetamine abusers is skin sores. Many users experience delusions of something crawling on or under their skin, and respond with aggressive skin picking or digging (10) (Figs. 11-7, 11-8).

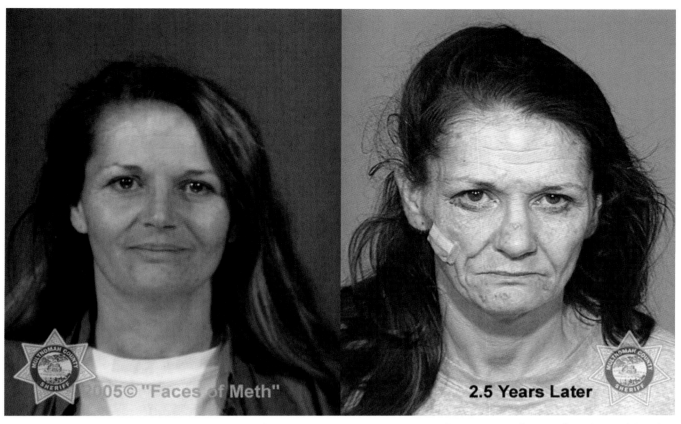

Figure 11-7: Change in appearance after methamphetamine use. From www.facesofmeth.us. Used with permission of Multnomah County Sheriff's Office, Portland, OR.

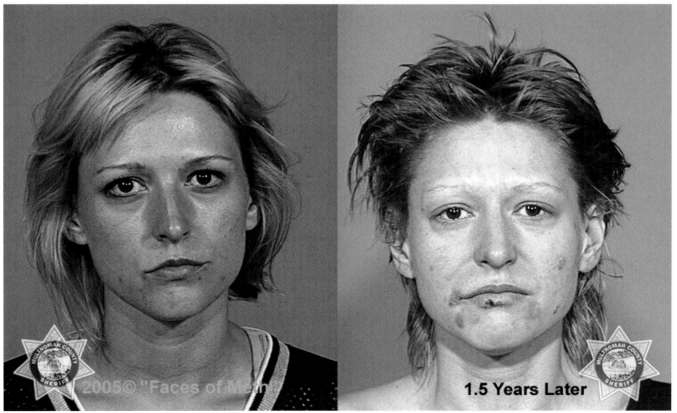

Figure 11-8: Change in appearance after methamphetamine use. From www.facesofmeth.us. Used with permission of Multnomah County Sheriff's Office, Portland, OR.

Methamphetamine use during pregnancy can cause premature birth, birth defects, and withdrawal symptoms in the newborn (5, 8).

Methamphetamine use is associated with the transmission of HIV and hepatitis through shared needles and high-risk sexual behavior (8). There is also evidence that the drug may increase viral replication and worsen the progression of HIV (8). Recovery from methamphetamine addiction can occur but is difficult. Abusers usually require extensive help from rehabilitation programs (8).

The damage inflicted by methamphetamine is not limited to those who abuse it. The production of this drug is very dangerous. About 15 percent of discovered meth labs are found after an explosion or fire. In some hospitals, one-third of admissions for burn injuries are due to meth lab accidents. Methamphetamine production gives rise to many toxic fumes that contaminate buildings and vehicles. Children living in the vicinity of a meth lab sometimes die from the exposure of these toxic substances. Clearly, methamphetamine is a lose-lose proposition for the entire community!

OPIATES

Our bodies produce natural opiates that help relieve pain and improve mood in certain circumstances. Ever wonder why you feel good after a long run or a good laugh? It is due to the release of one type of these peptides called endorphins (13). Opiate drugs bind to the same opiate receptors in the brain as the endogenous opiates. Many of these drugs, including morphine, oxycodone, hydromorphone (Dilaudid), hydrocodone (Vicodin), codeine, meperidine (Demerol), and fentanyl, are some of the best painkillers in medicine. Others, such as heroin, are produced mainly to sell on the street to drug abusers seeking a high (Figs. 11-9, 11-10).

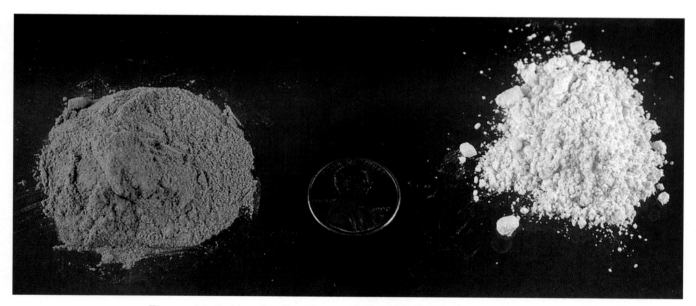

Figure 11-9: Heroin: Southeast Asian (R) Southwest Asian (L).
Photo courtesy of the Drug Enforcement Administration.

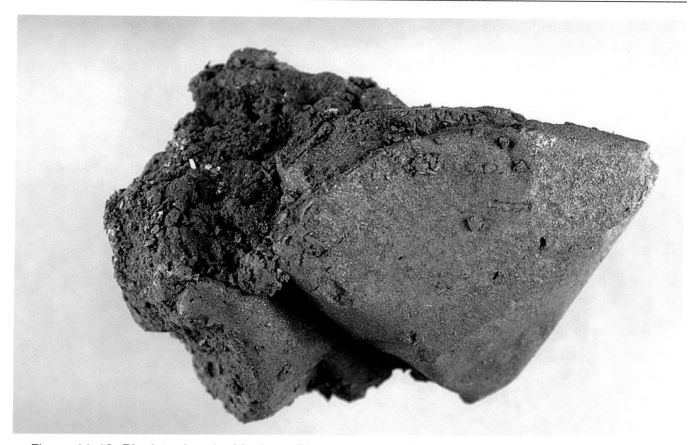

Figure 11-10: Black tar heroin, Mexican. Photo courtesy of the Drug Enforcement Administration.

Unfortunately, abuse of all types of opiate drugs is common in the United States. Each year, more than 2 million teenagers abuse prescription pain relievers such as Vicodin and Oxycontin (14). Every day, 2,500 American youth (ages twelve to seventeen) abuse a prescription pain reliever for the first time (14). A 2008 national survey on drug use estimated that 3.8 million Americans had used heroin at some point in their lives, and over 450,000 had used it in the past year (1).

Opiates may be swallowed, injected intravenously, or inhaled. Abusers use the drug to get a surge of pleasurable sensation called a rush. Intravenous injection provides the most intense rush and is often the preferred route of administration in experienced users (15). However, the side effects of opiate abuse quickly outweigh any benefit. Some of the first side effects seen include drowsiness and clouded mental function for several hours. Cardiac function and breathing are slowed. The respiratory depression that accompanies opiate use accounts for most of the acute deaths associated with their use. Chronic use often results in tolerance, and larger doses of the drug are needed to get the desired effect.

The uncertainty of the concentration of drugs bought on the street, along with tolerance, often leads to overdose, which can cause seizures, respiratory arrest, and death (5). Intravenous drug use is associated with serious infections of the skin, heart valves, liver, and lungs. One study of opiate addicts who had been admitted to the hospital found that more than 10 percent had endocarditis, an infection of the heart valves (5). From shared needles, intravenous drug users are also prone to develop infections such as hepatitis B, hepatitis C, and HIV/AIDS. About 70 to 80 percent of new hepatitis C infections in the US each year are thought to be due to intravenous drug use (15).

Chronic abuse leads to addiction. If an addict stops using the drug, withdrawal symptoms such as drug craving, restlessness, muscle and bone pain, insomnia, diarrhea, vomiting, cold flashes, yawning, and abdominal cramps develop (15, 16). Once addicted, the abuser's primary purpose in life often becomes finding and using drugs. Family, friends, and jobs fall to the wayside.

Treatment to overcome addiction involves supportive care and medications to help minimize withdrawal symptoms (16). Support groups such as Narcotics Anonymous (www.na.org) and SMART Recovery (www.smartrecovery.org) can be very helpful (16).

MARIJUANA

Marijuana (Figs. 11-11, 11-12) is a mixture of shredded dry parts of the hemp plant Cannabis sativa (17). It is the most commonly used illicit drug in America, with an estimated 102 million US citizens (41 percent of the population) having tried the drug at least once (1).

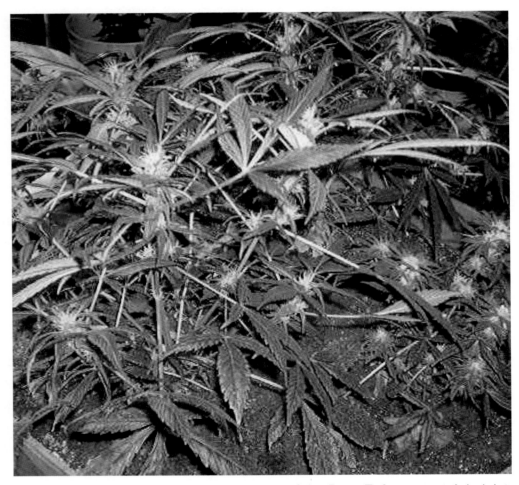

Figure 11-11: Marijuana plants. Photo courtesy of the Drug Enforcement Administration.

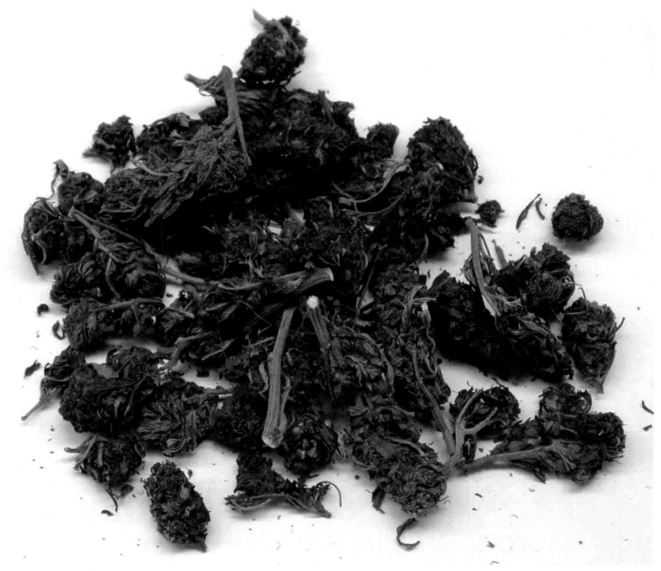

Figure 11-12: Dried marijuana. Photo courtesy of the Drug Enforcement Administration.

Marijuana is usually smoked, but it is also blended with foods or used to make a tea (17). Its main mind-altering chemical is delta-9-tetrahydrocannabinol, or THC. THC appears to affect the hippocampus, a part of the brain associated with memory (17). Short-term effects include impaired memory and learning, distorted perception, loss of coordination, increased heart rate, and anxiety (17). Chronic use is associated with impaired learning, poor memory, anxiety, depression, suicidal thoughts, and schizophrenia (17). Studies of students with similar standardized test scores in the fourth grade showed that students who went on to become regular marijuana smokers had significantly lower test scores in the twelfth grade compared to those of nonsmokers (17). Studies of college students found that heavy marijuana users suffered from impaired learning, poor memory, and inattention, even if they had not used the drug within the past twenty-four hours (17).

As if that weren't reason enough to stay away from pot, marijuana smoke may also cause lung injury similar to tobacco smoke. A recent study found that smoking marijuana more than fifty times over the course of your life doubles your risk of lung cancer (19).

Long-term marijuana use can lead to physical dependence and addiction (17). Withdrawal symptoms include drug craving, irritability, decreased appetite, insomnia, and anxiety (17). While the withdrawal symptoms from quitting marijuana are often milder than those associated with cocaine or heroin abuse, they can be significant. You can find free help at Marijuana Addiction Help (www.marijuana-addict.com) and SMART Recovery (www.smartrecovery.org).

INHALANTS

Many chemicals found in hundreds of different household products have been inhaled for mind-altering effects. Some of these products include paint thinners or removers, dry-cleaning fluids, correction fluids, gasoline, felt-tip markers, spray paint, hair sprays, deodorant aerosols, cooking sprays, fabric protectors, ether, chloroform, nitrous oxide, butane lighters, propane, whipped cream dispensers, and various nitrites referred to as "poppers," such as amyl nitrite, isobutyl nitrite, and isopropyl nitrite (18). It is estimated that over 22 million Americans have used inhalants, with 2 million using them in 2008 (1). Use of inhalants is especially common among young people. One study found that over 15 percent of eighth-graders reported previous inhalant use (18).

Most inhalants can produce a state similar to alcohol intoxication. Prolonged sniffing can produce a loss of sensation, unconsciousness, irregular heart rhythm, and death (18). The syndrome known as "sudden sniffing death" can occur within minutes of a single session of inhalant use (18). Chronic use can damage the heart, lungs, kidneys, and liver, and addiction associated with relatively mild withdrawal symptoms can also occur (18).

PERSONAL OBSERVATIONS

As a surgical pathologist, I saw many cases of hepatitis and AIDS caused by drug abuse. My colleagues in clinical medicine and forensic pathology had it much worse. They had to endure seeing many healthy young people die directly from drug abuse. The tragic loss of health and lives from drug abuse can be totally eliminated by lifestyle choices. The health risks of abusing drugs far outweigh any possible benefits. Anyone who encourages you to abuse drugs is not acting in your best interest. *Just say no!*

REFERENCES:

1. Substance Abuse and Mental Health Services Administration. "Results from the 2008 National Survey on Drug Use and Health: National Findings." Rockville, MD: Office of Applied Studies, 2009. NSDUH Series H-36, HHS Publication No. SMA 09-4434.

2. Mokdad et al. "Actual Causes of Death in the United States, 2000." *Journal of the American Medical Association*, 291 (2004): 1238, 1240.

3. Kassed et al. "Hospitalizations Related to Drug Abuse, 2005." Agency for Healthcare Research and Quality. Rockville, MD, October 2007. HCUP Statistical Brief #39.

4. Office of National Drug Control Policy. "Drug-Related Crime." Drug Policy Information Clearinghouse Fact Sheet. Washington, DC: ONDCP, March 2000.

5. Kane AB, Kumar V. "Environmental and Nutritional Pathology." In *Robbins and Cotran Pathologic Basis of Disease*, 7th ed., edited by Kumar et al, 419–28. Philadelphia, PA: Elsevier Saunders, 2005.

6. Cocaine, Marijuana, and Heroin Have Highest Rates of U.S. Emergency Department Illicit Drug-Related Visits. CESAR FAX. (A Weekly FAX from the Center for Substance Abuse Research) Vol. 22, Issue 38 , September 23, 2013.

7. National Institute on Drug Abuse. "NIDA InfoFacts: Cocaine." Bethesda, MD: NIDA, March 8, 2010. www.drugabuse.gov.

8. National Institute on Drug Abuse. "Methamphetamine—Abuse and Addiction." Bethesda, MD: NIDA, September 2006. NIH Publication Number 06-4210.

9. National Institute on Drug Abuse. "Methamphetamine Addiction: Cause for Concern—Hope for the Future." Bethesda, MD: NIDA, March 2007.

10. Center for Substance Abuse Research (CESAR). "Methamphetamine." University of Maryland, October 18, 2005. cesar.umd.edu.

11. Davey M. "Dental Problems from Methamphetamine: Grisly Effect of One Drug: 'Meth Mouth.'" *New York Times*. June 11, 2005.

12. Meth Awareness and Prevention Project of South Dakota (MAPP-SD). "Ingredients in Meth." www.mappsd.org.

13. Walker M. "Endorphins 101: Your Guide to Natural Euphoria." June 29, 2006. www.ivillage.com.

14. Office of National Drug Control Policy. "Prescription for Danger—A Report on the Troubling Trend of Prescription and Over-the-Counter Drug Abuse among the Nation's Teens." Washington, DC: ONDCP, January 2008.

15. Office of National Drug Control Policy. "Heroin Facts & Figures." Washington, DC: ONDCP, April 2010.

16. Medline Plus, a service of the US National Library of Medicine and the National Institutes of Health. "Opiate Withdrawal." April 20, 2009. http://www.nlm.nih.gov/medlineplus/ency/article/000949.htm.

17. Office of National Drug Control Policy. "Marijuana Facts & Figures." Washington, DC: ONDCP, April 2010.

18. Office of National Drug Control Policy. "Inhalants Facts & Figures." Washington, DC: ONDCP, April 2010.

19. Callaghan et al. "Marijuana Use and Risk of Lung Cancer: A 40-Year Cohort Study." *Cancer Causes and Control* 10 (October 24, 2013): 1811–20.

20. What is the scope of methamphetamine abuse in the United States? NIDA Research Report Series. Last updated September 2013.

PART III
PREVENTION

12: EXERCISE

Physical exercise is one of the most effective ways to decrease your chances of disease. An age-adjusted mortality study of over 6,000 healthy men was performed after dividing the men into five groups based on their fitness levels. The death rate of the least fit group was 4.5 times the death rate of the most fit group (1, 2). Even at age fifty, starting and maintaining an exercise program increases life expectancy as much as if you were to quit smoking (3). Exercise can help prevent some of the most deadly diseases in our society, including atherosclerosis, obesity, diabetes, and cancer (2, 4). Exercise can also improve quality of life and affords important mental benefits, such as a lower risk of dementia, decreased incidence of depression, relief of mental stress, and increased self-esteem (4, 7).

Despite all of these benefits, less than one-third of Americans exercise enough to meet the minimal activity levels recommended by national organizations such as the American Heart Association and the Centers for Disease Control and Prevention (2). The current recommendations are two hours and thirty minutes of moderate aerobic exercise (such as brisk walking) per week and two strength-building activities per week that work all major muscle groups. It is estimated that up to 250,000 deaths per year in the US are due to a lack of regular exercise (2).

Exercise helps prevent atherosclerosis by lowering blood pressure, decreasing triglycerides, decreasing total cholesterol, decreasing low-density (bad) lipoproteins, and increasing high-density (good) lipoproteins (2). The calories burned during exercise help prevent and reverse obesity and its many complications. Exercise improves insulin sensitivity and can help prevent or reverse type 2 diabetes (2, 4). Vigorous exercisers are also 30 percent less likely to develop breast cancer and 30 to 40 percent less likely to develop colon cancer (5, 6). The mechanisms behind these benefits of exercise are not well established and continue to be studied.

Three components to physical exercise contribute to our health. Most of the systemic effects described above are stimulated most by aerobic, or endurance, exercises such as walking, running, swimming, or biking. Resistance exercises such as weight training develop muscle strength, strengthen bones and ligaments, and help prevent musculoskeletal problems such as low back pain. Stretching exercises increase flexibility and contribute to better physical function and injury prevention. These three components are described in more detail throughout this chapter.

AEROBIC EXERCISES

The US Department of Health and Human Services recommends at least 150 minutes of moderate-intensity aerobic exercise each week for good health (8). More is better, but any is better than none (8). Any type of sustained endurance activity is beneficial. Walking is a highly recommended activity, especially for individuals who are just beginning an exercise program. Jogging, running, swimming, biking, dancing, and hiking are all excellent activities, as are climbing stairs and becoming active in sports. Even active chores, such as pushing a lawn mower or chopping wood, can have benefits in terms of maintaining your health.

The key to success is to incorporate exercise into your daily lifestyle. Look for activities that are enjoyable and easy to work into your day. An exercise program that you find unpleasant, disruptive to your schedule, or overly expensive is not likely to succeed. Look for ways to exercise with minimal waste of time and money.

Often, exercise can be incorporated into another activity you already have in your schedule.

A walk with family or friends can be both social recreation and beneficial exercise. Using a push lawn mower rather than a rider allows you to cut the lawn and work out at the same time. Use of stationary exercise machines, such as a stepping block (Fig. 12-1), treadmill, or stationary bike, allows one to exercise while watching television. Habits such as taking stairs instead of elevators, and walking or biking instead of a short car ride, are other easy ways to incorporate exercise into your daily routine.

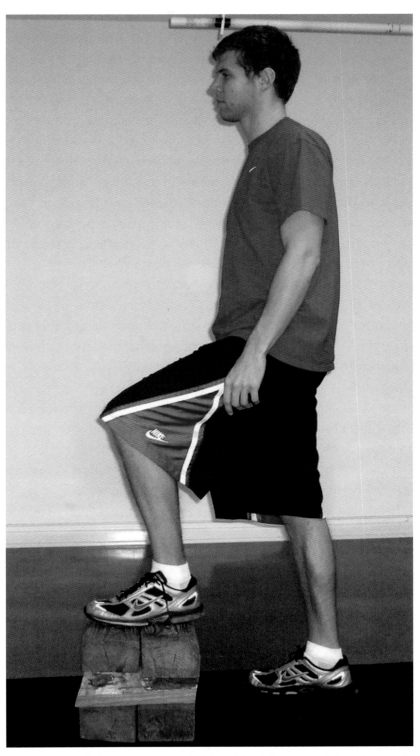

Figure 12-1: Stepping up and down on any stable object is a good low-impact aerobic exercise.

When starting any aerobic exercise routine, remember to take it slow and easy. Running to exhaustion on the first day will likely make you so sore that you will be tempted to quit. Start slow, and gradually increase exercise time and intensity as your fitness level increases.

RESISTANCE (STRENGTH) TRAINING

Whereas endurance training involves exercising against low resistance for a relatively long period of time in order to strengthen the heart, resistance training involves exercising with heavy resistance for a short period of time to develop skeletal muscle strength. The terms "repetitions (reps)" and "sets" are used to describe strength-training routines. Resistance exercises are usually performed until failure, which in this case is defined as the inability to do the exercise any longer while maintaining good form. A repetition is the act of performing a given exercise one time. A set is a group of repetitions done without an intervening rest period. For example, if you do ten push-ups without stopping, you have done one set of ten repetitions. The American Heart Association recommends at least eight to ten sets of resistance exercises—at least one for each major muscle group—twice a week to build muscle strength (4).

Muscle groups that control opposing movements are called antagonistic muscles. Examples of these include muscles of the chest and upper back, triceps and biceps in the arm, quadriceps and hamstrings in the leg, and the abdominal and lower back muscles of the trunk. Development of one major muscle group without similar development of the corresponding antagonistic muscle group can lead to imbalances, and predispose you to injury or poor posture.

Effective strength training can be accomplished at home using very little equipment, or at a gym with the latest high-tech gadgetry. The path you choose is a matter of personal preference. Again, making it easy and fun is the key to success. In general, it is desirable to mainly include exercises that use simple calisthenics or free weights rather than complex machines that overly isolate muscle groups. This is because exercising with free weights or calisthenics develop stabilizing core muscles as well as the primary muscles targeted.

For example, when you do squats, you are exercising your lower back as well as your legs, and doing a movement that more closely resembles lifting objects in daily life. In contrast, using a seated leg-press machine only exercises your legs. However, such machines can be very valuable in certain instances. If you are recovering from strained back muscles, the seated leg-press machine allows you to work out your legs while resting your back. A common mistake for beginners is to try too much too fast. This usually results in painful consequences and can sometimes lead to serious injury. Take it slow, make it fun, and keep at it!

The following section outlines some of my favorite strength exercises that can be performed at home as well as at the gym. In general, I recommend doing ten to fifteen repetitions per set. Exercises are organized according to the muscle groups targeted.

CHEST

The powerful pectoral muscles of the chest are used to pull your arms toward the center of your body or push things away from you. These movements are common in our daily activities.

PUSH-UPS

This familiar exercise develops the chest as well as the front of the shoulders and the triceps. Place your hands approximately shoulder-width apart and lower your body until your chest touches the floor; push up until your elbows are locked (Fig. 12-2). If you find it difficult to do ten push-ups in a set, try kneeling push-ups, where your knees rather than your toes touch the floor (Fig. 12-3). A more advanced variation that allows a fuller range of motion and stretching of the pectoral muscles is an elevated push-up, where blocks are placed under your hands (Fig. 12-4).

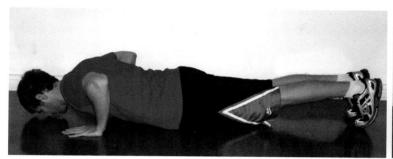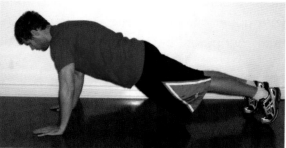

Figure 12-2: Push-up.

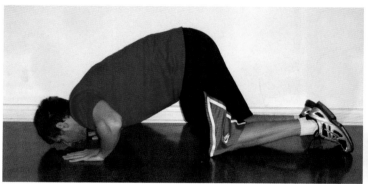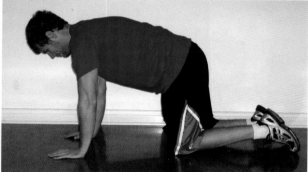

Figure 12-3: Kneeling push-up.

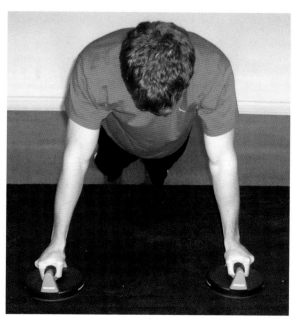

Figure 12-4: Elevated push-up. The use of some type of extender, such as the Perfect Pushup product shown here, allows push-ups with an increased range of motion.

BENCH PRESSES

The motion used in bench presses is similar to a push-up except you lie on your back and press a barbell (Fig. 12-5). If heavy weights are used, it is important to have a training partner spot you; otherwise, a missed repetition can leave you trapped under the bar—a dangerous predicament to be in, especially if you're a beginner. Some weight benches are adjustable, which allows variations of the bench press. Inclined bench presses are performed with your head elevated above your pelvis. This exercise works your upper chest and anterior shoulder. Declined bench presses are performed with your head lower than your pelvis; their purpose is to help develop your lower pectoral muscles.

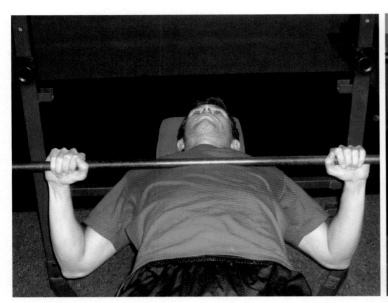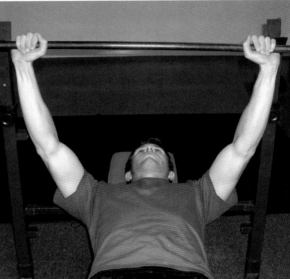

Figure 12-5: Bench press.

DUMBBELL FLIES

Dumbbell flies are an excellent exercise that stretches and develops your pectoral muscles. Lie on your back with dumbbells extended over your body. Lower them with your arms bent as far as you can (Fig. 12-6) and return the weight to the original position. The movement is similar to hugging a large tree. At the lower position, keep the dumbbells as far apart as possible, and resist the temptation to move your elbows.

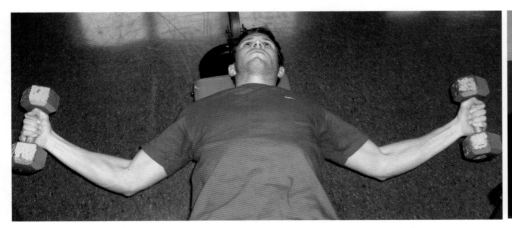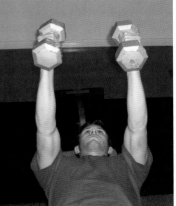

Figure 12-6: Dumbbell flies.

UPPER BACK

The upper back muscles are antagonistic to the chest muscles. If they are not developed to the same extent as the pectoral muscles, the shoulders tend to be pulled forward, ruining your posture. For this reason, many like to exercise the upper back on the same days as they work their chest.

SHOULDER SHRUGS

This is an excellent exercise to develop the trapezius of your upper back. Stand straight, with a relatively heavy dumbbell in each hand. Shrug your shoulders as high as you can and then return them to the resting position (Fig. 12-7).

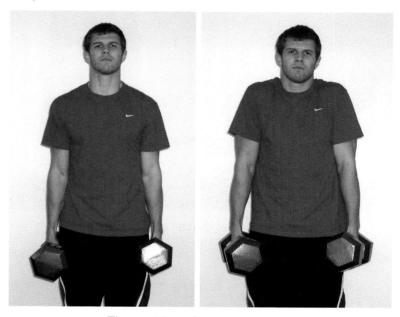

Figure 12-7: Shoulder shrug.

DUMBBELL ROWS

Support your body with one hand on a bench or chair and use the other to lift a dumbbell in an arching movement (Fig. 12-8). This movement will also exercise your upper arm, but concentrate on using your back muscles as you complete each row. Repeat the movement for an equal number of repetitions using the other arm.

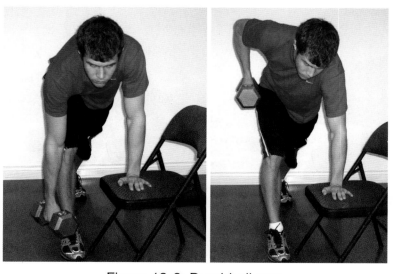

Figure 12-8: Dumbbell row.

BENT-OVER LATERAL RAISES

This exercise is like dumbbell flies in reverse. Bend over with your head level with your hips. Start with your arms straight and your hands together. Raise your hands to the side until they are level with your shoulders (Fig. 12-9). You don't need a lot of weight for this exercise. Two cans of vegetables may provide enough weight at first.

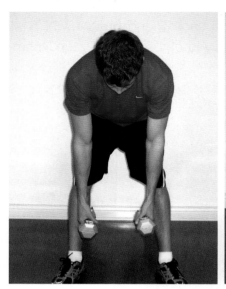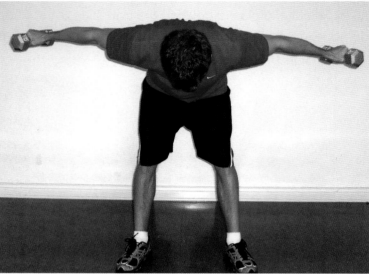

Figure 12-9: Bent-over lateral raises.

SPRING PULLS

For some reason, this spring device is commonly called a chest expander. However, it is most valuable for exercising the upper back. This exercise is similar to bent-over lateral raises except that using the spring allows you to stand up straight. This is an excellent exercise for developing the rhomboids between your shoulder blades. These muscles pull the arms in the opposite direction of your pectoral muscles. You may be able to use more resistance if you hold the spring high and allow the large latissimus muscles on the sides of your back to do most of the work. However, it is best to keep the spring below your chest and concentrate on using your upper back muscles (Fig. 12-10).

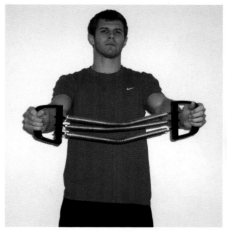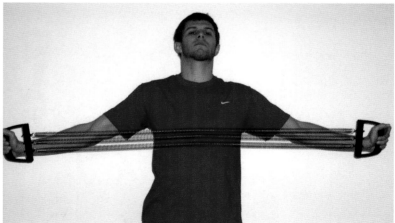

Figure 12-10: Spring pulls.

PULL-UPS

Pull-ups (Fig. 12-11) are an excellent all-around back conditioner but emphasize the development of the large muscles of the sides of your back called latissimus dorsi. These muscles have antagonistic movements more directly opposed to the shoulders than the chest. Some may prefer to do this exercise in combination with shoulder workouts. A relatively wide grip emphasizes back development, while keeping your hands closer together on the bar targets the biceps. If you find conventional pull-ups too difficult, try using a chair to assist you (Fig. 12-12).

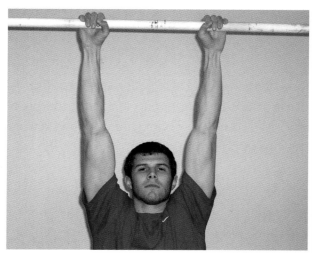 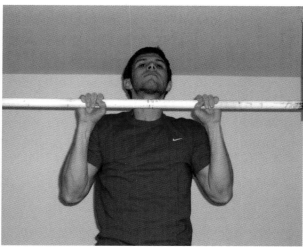

Figure 12-11: Pull-up.

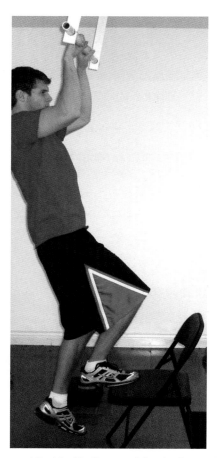

Figure 12-12: Pull-up with chair assist.

ABDOMINAL MUSCLES

Abdominal muscles are very important in our routine daily activities. As part of our core muscles, they help form a link facilitating power transfer between the lower and upper body. Almost all complex movements from hitting a tennis ball to carrying a bag of groceries engage the abdominal muscles. They are critical in maintaining balance and good posture. With the lower back muscles, they help support the spinal column. Low back pain effects 80 percent of Americans at some point of their lives and weak abdominal muscles is one of the major factors contributing to this painful debilitating condition. Time spent in strengthening the abdominal muscles is a good investment.

SIT-UPS

This familiar exercise is best performed with your knees bent and your feet flat on the floor (Fig. 12-13). Avoid putting your hands behind your head and pulling forward, as this can lead to neck problems. Placing your hands under your hips will prevent you from rubbing your backside raw, and can reduce the temptation to use your arms instead of your abdomen to pull you forward.

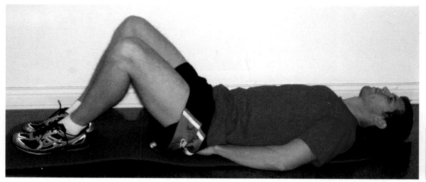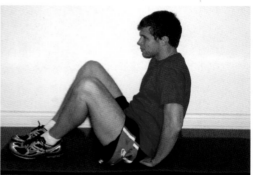

Figure 12-13: Sit-up.

LEG LIFTS

Lying flat on your back with your legs extended, raise your legs to a vertical position before slowly returning them to the floor (Fig. 12-14).

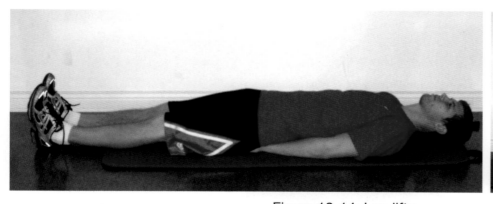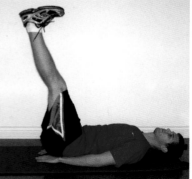

Figure 12-14: Leg lifts.

PELVIC THRUST

First, do a leg lift. Then, instead of lowering your legs, raise your hips off the floor like you are attempting to touch your heels to the ceiling (Fig. 12-15).

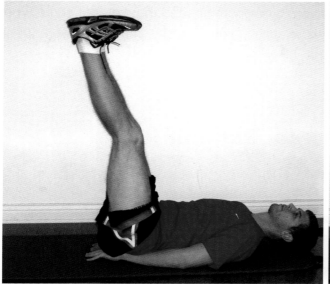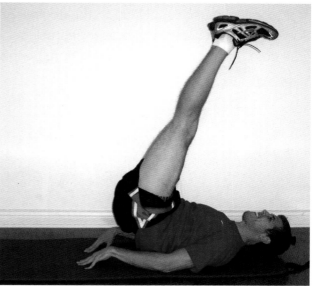

Figure 12-15: Pelvic thrust.

LEG LIFT THRUSTS

This very effective exercise is performed like leg lifts except the pelvis is lifted by the abdominal muscles in the top position like a pelvic thrust.

CRUNCHES

This exercise is a combination of sit-ups and leg lifts. Lie on your back and place your hands under your buttocks to reduce friction. Now raise your upper body and legs at the same time (Fig. 12-16).

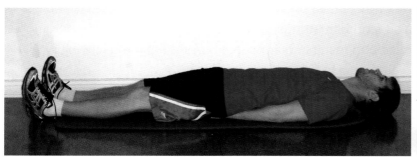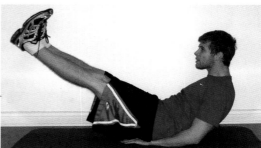

Figure 12-16: Crunches.

AB ROLLER

This is a simple and highly effective high-resistance abdominal workout. The ab wheel required for this workout is inexpensive and can be purchased at most stores with a sporting goods department. From a kneeling position, roll the wheel out until you are prone with your arms extended (Fig. 12-17). Then, using your abdominal muscles, pull up to the original position. It is recommended that you put some type of padding under your knees to prevent abrasions. This relatively high-intensity abdominal workout also targets core muscles, the lower chest, and the triceps.

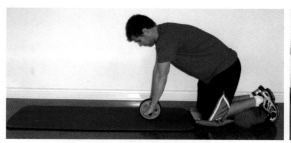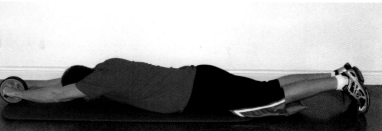

Figure 12-17: Ab roller.

LOWER BACK

Like the abdominal muscles, the lower back muscles are a major component of the core muscles that are involved in many daily activities, balance, and posture. The muscles of the lower back are particularly important in supporting the spine. A strong lower back is a good defense against lower back injury and pain. It is a good idea to develop the lower back in concert with the abdominal muscles. Strong abdominal muscles and weak lower back muscles can lead to poor posture and injury. <u>Go slowly when starting lower back strength-building exercises. Doing too much too fast can lead to painful back spasms and serious injury.</u>

GOOD-MORNING EXERCISE

From a standing position, bend forward at the waist ninety degrees and use your lower back to return upright (Fig. 12-18). This exercise targets the muscles of the lower back and back of the legs, including the erector spinae muscles, gluteus muscles, and hamstrings. Use low resistance and high repetitions; using heavy weights while doing this exercise can result in blackouts and/or painful muscle injury.

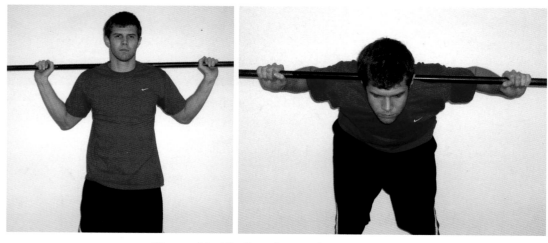

Figure 12-18: Good-morning exercise.

SHOULDERS

The shoulder is a complex joint that allows a wide variety of movements. Shoulder muscles are involved any time you move the upper arm up, down, forward, backward or sideways. They play a major role when you throw a ball, swim or play tennis. Unfortunately injuries to shoulder muscles are common, painful and debilitating. Strengthening the shoulder muscles will go a long way in helping to prevent shoulder injuries. While the chest and upper back exercises listed above will help develop the front and back of the shoulder, the exercises listed below will help strengthen the rest of the shoulder muscles.

MILITARY PRESS

This exercise can be performed with either a barbell or dumbbells (Fig. 12-19). Starting with the weight on your shoulders, lift the weight overhead and return. This is a particularly good exercise for the deltoids, triceps, and stabilizing muscles of the trunk.

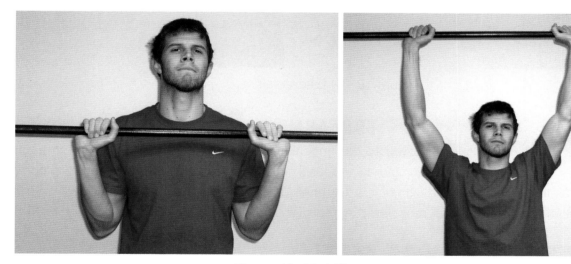

Figure 12-19: Military press.

DECLINE PUSH-UPS

This is one of the few good shoulder exercises that doesn't require weights. It is performed like a push-up but with your feet elevated. The result? Your shoulders do more of the work (Fig. 12-20). The higher your feet, the more your shoulders are isolated.

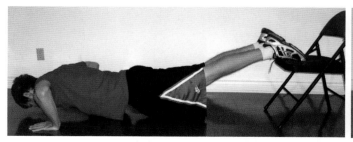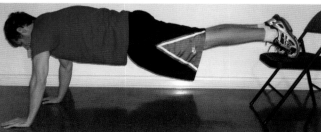

Figure 12-20: Decline push-ups.

LATERAL RAISES

Using light weights and keeping your arms extended, lift the weights from your side to slightly above your shoulder (Fig. 12-21). This exercise works the side of the deltoid. It is especially effective if your hands are slightly tilted downward, with the little finger higher than the thumb.

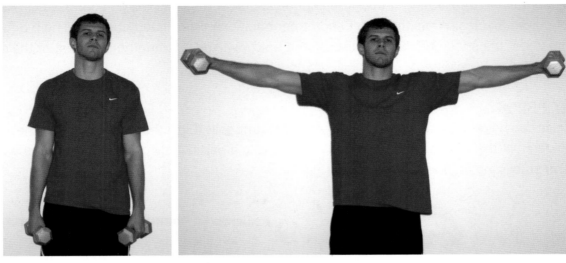

Figure 12-21: Lateral raises.

FOREARMS

The muscles of the forearm supply power to the fingers and wrists. They give us the grip strength to hang from a bar and enable us to open a screw top jar. These muscles also play a major role in complex motions such as throwing a ball and swinging a bat (ever wonder why many baseball players have huge forearms?). Developing the forearm muscles can improve our quality of life and help prevent injury.

HAND GRIPPERS/GRIPPING BALLS

One of the most common exercises used to develop the flexors of the hand and fingers is to squeeze a ball or hand gripper (Fig. 12-22). The muscles controlling the thumb can also be exercised by pressing the thumb toward the fingers (Fig. 12-23).

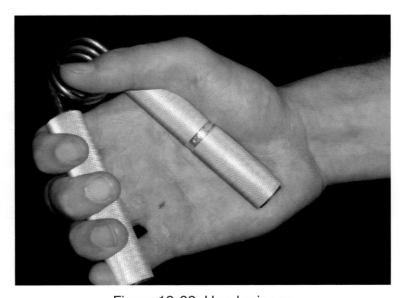

Figure 12-22: Hand gripper.

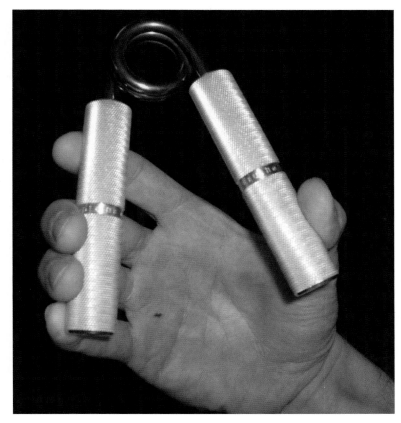

Figure 12-23: Thumb flexor exercise.

WRIST CURLS

Sit on a chair or bench with your arms over your knees, and flex the weight upward moving only your wrists (Fig. 12-24). This exercise can be used with a barbell or dumbbells, and a variation of this exercise can be done by extending and flexing your fingers (Fig. 12-25).

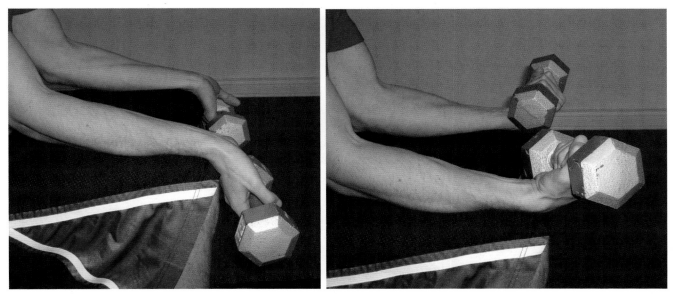

Figure 12-24: Wrist curl.

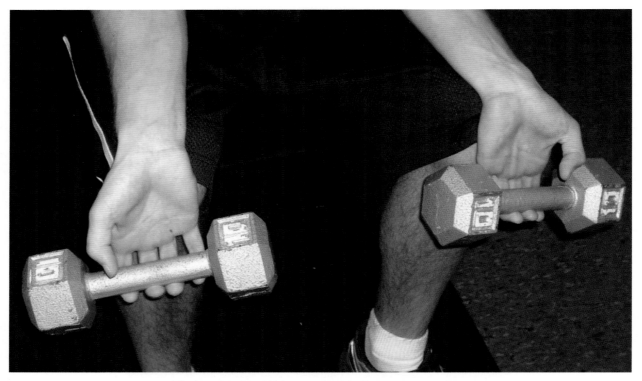

Figure 12-25: Wrist curl with finger extension.

REVERSE WRIST CURLS

Similar to wrist curls, reverse wrist curls are done with your palms down instead of up (Fig. 12-26). This helps develop the muscles of your forearm between the back of your hand and your elbow.

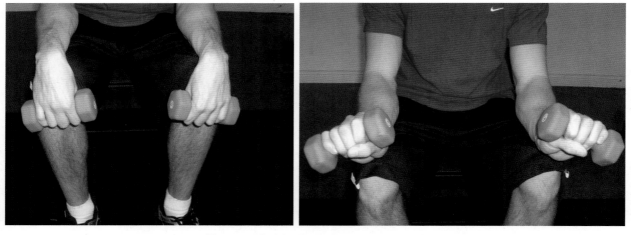

Figure 12-26: Reverse wrist curls.

LEGS

Leg muscles are our main source of power for locomotion. They are used in everyday activies such as walking, squatting, and getting up from a chair. They are critical to most sports, allowing us to run and jump. Strong leg muscles also support the knee, ankle, and hip joints helping to prevent injury. Strong legs can help prevent falls as we get older. Time spent developing the leg muscles will help our quality of life at any age.

SQUATS

Squats (Fig. 12-27) are one of the most effective exercises for developing your upper leg and lower back. Begin by placing the barbell on a squat rack. Position yourself under the weight, with the bar lying across your shoulders. While keeping your upper body relatively straight and upright, bend your knees into the squat position.

In general, it is safer to only go about halfway down to horizontal. Complete the movement by using your leg muscles to stand up again. Heavy squats are dangerous if performed alone without safeguards. Have training partners spot you to prevent injury in case you lose your balance or fail a repetition. Many gyms also have an enclosure called a squat cage that will catch the weight if you are unable to complete a repetition. If heavy weights are used, there is a tendency for your shoulders to become bruised. This can be prevented by using a padding device such as the Manta Ray (Fig. 12-28).

High repetitions of squat exercises without weights can also provide a good leg workout. Use a broomstick or non-weighted bar to increase your stability.

Wall squats are an excellent exercise, and you don't even need weights. With your back against the wall, lower yourself into the squat position (Fig. 12-29) and hold until it burns. Once you can do this for sixty seconds easily, try doing wall squats with only one leg.

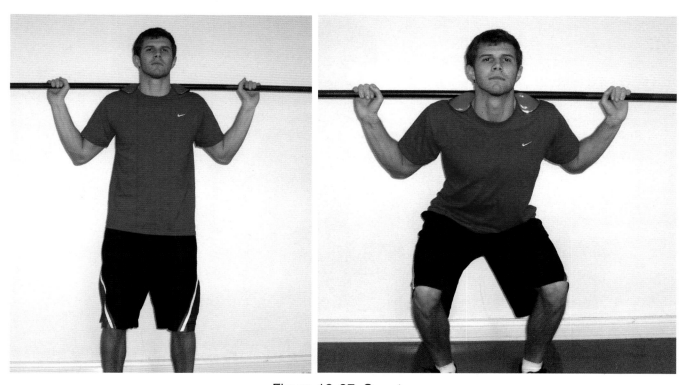

Figure 12-27: Squats.

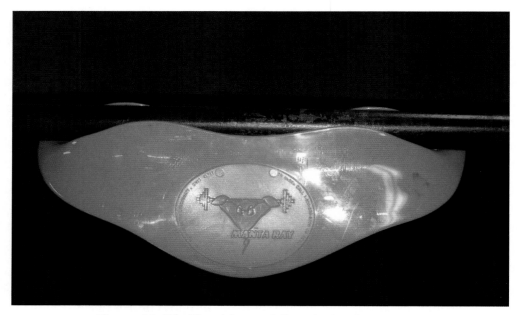

Figure 12-28: Shoulder padding device for squats.

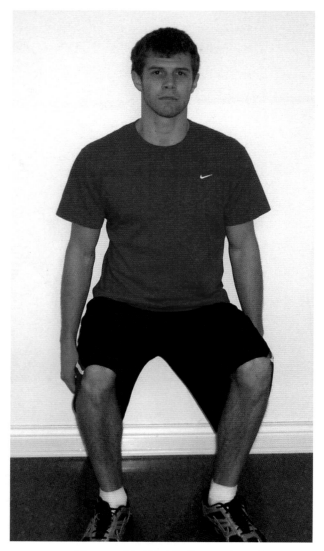

Figure 12-29: Wall squats.

CALF RAISES

This exercise targets your calves, including the gastrocnemius and soleus muscles. Stand on some sort of block, such as an old telephone book, so you can simultaneously stretch your calf muscles by allowing your heel to drop below horizontal (Fig. 12-30). Hold on to a pull-up bar, wall, or chair to maintain your balance. When this exercise becomes easy, try it with one leg. When one-legged calf raises become easy, try holding a dumbbell in your free hand.

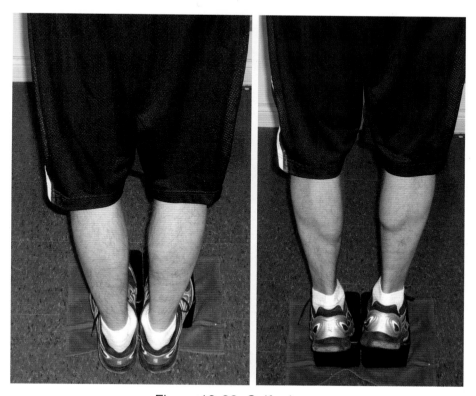

Figure 12-30: Calf raises.

ONE-LEG LUNGES

One-leg lunges are an excellent upper leg exercise that can be performed without weights (Fig. 12-31) or by using a dumbbell. Most people will benefit from using a chair to help maintain balance.

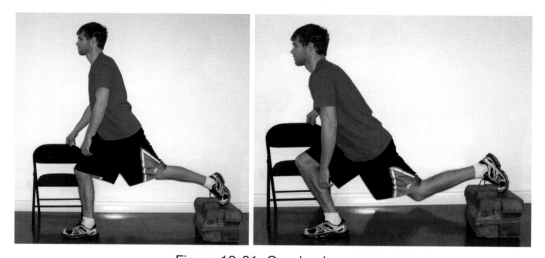

Figure 12-31: One-leg lunges.

SUPER SKATERS

Super skaters are another excellent leg exercise that doesn't require weights. Keeping one foot off the floor, make speed-skating motions to exercise the opposite leg (Fig. 12-32). A chair can be used to help maintain balance.

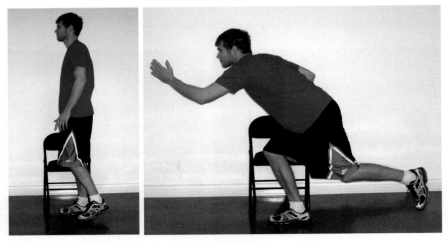

Figure 12-32: Super skaters.

ARMS

The major muscles of the upper arm are the biceps, which flex your arm at the elbow, and the triceps, which extend your arm at the elbow. These muscles are used almost every time we move something with our hands.

CURLS

There are many variations of curls that develop the biceps (Fig. 12-33 to Fig. 12-37). Doing standard curls with a straight bar can lead you to strain the ulnar side of the wrist (in other words, the pinky-finger side); doing this exercise with a bent curl bar or dumbbells is recommended. Besides flexing the arm, the biceps are also the muscle that rotates the forearm and hand so that the thumb points away from the body. This movement is called supination and is used when we open a screw-top lid on a jar. Incorporation of a supination movement into the curl exercises can be accomplished by starting with your thumb forward and ending with your palms up (Fig. 12-35).

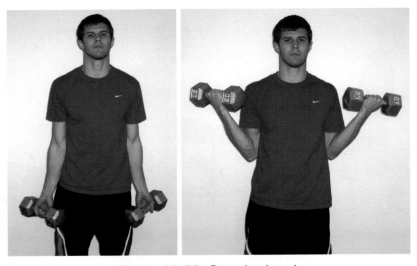

Figure 12-33: Standard curl.

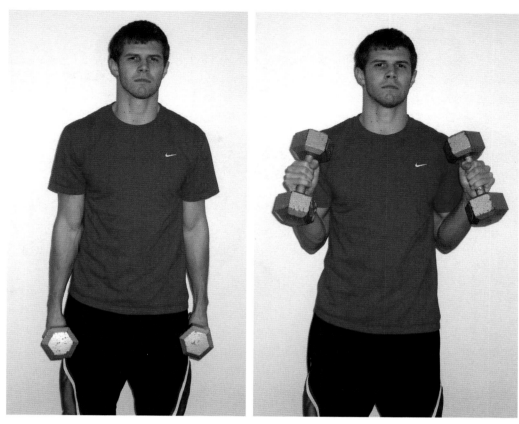

Figure 12-34: Hammer curls (thumbs forward).

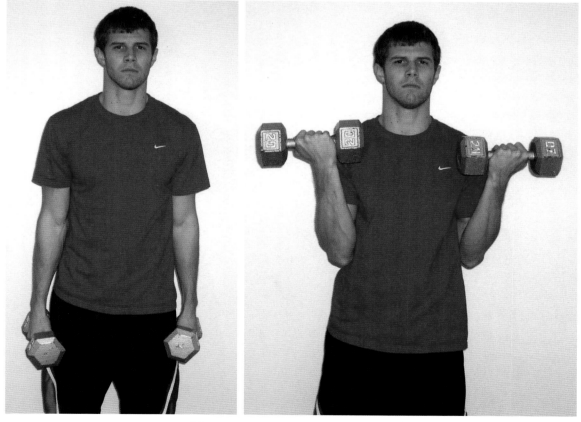

Figure 12-35: Supination curls.

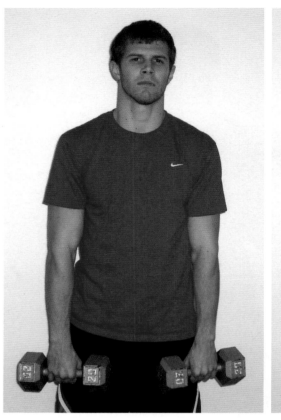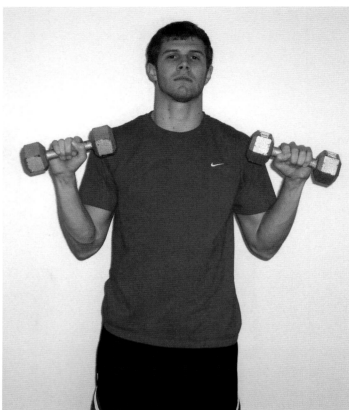

Figure 12-36: Reverse curls (palms down).

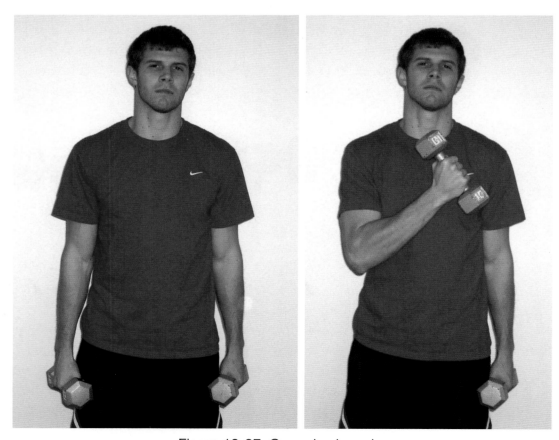

Figure 12-37: Cross-body curls.

DUMBBELL TRICEP PRESSES

For this exercise, lie on the floor or a bench with dumbbells in hand and your elbows pointed toward the ceiling. Lower the weight adjacent to your ear and then press your arms up straight (Fig. 12-38). In all triceps exercises, it is important to keep your elbows parallel to the body. Rotating your elbows out can lead to injury.

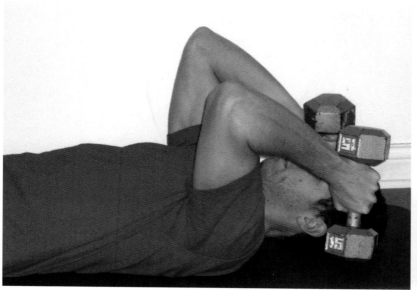
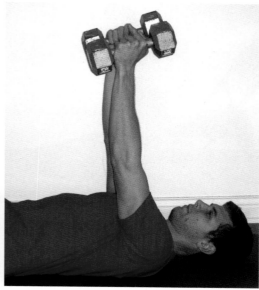

Figure 12-38: Tricep presses.

STANDING TRICEP PRESSES (FRENCH CURL)

This exercise has the same movement as the dumbbell triceps press but is performed in a standing position (Fig. 12-39). Use of dumbbells or a specially made triceps press bar is recommended. Using a standard straight barbell makes it difficult to keep your elbows in, which makes you vulnerable to elbow injury.

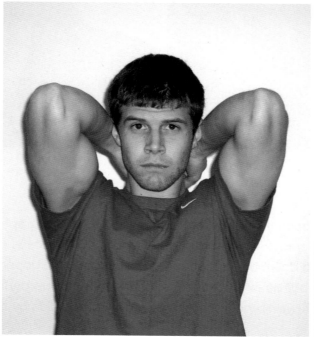
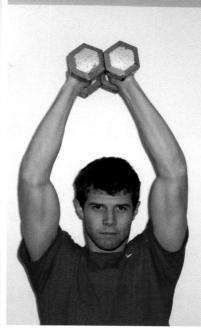

Figure 12-39: Standing tricep presses.

DIPS

This is a good exercise for your triceps and lower chest, and requires no weights. Leaning against a bench or chair, lower and raise your body moving only your elbow joint (Fig. 12-40).

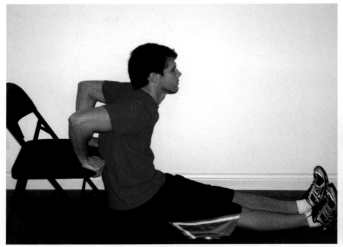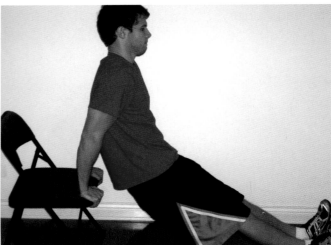

Figure 12-40: Dips.

SIDE TRICEP RAISES

This is a great triceps exercise that requires no weights. Lie on your left side with your right hand on the floor under your armpit and your left hand on your right shoulder. Raise your upper body by extending your right arm (Fig. 12-41). Lower back down and repeat. After you finish a set, turn over and repeat with the opposite arm. I recommend using a padded mat to avoid hip bruises.

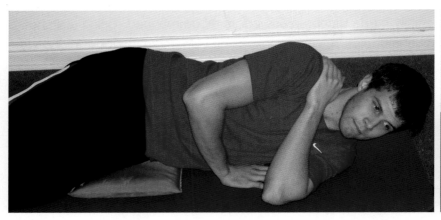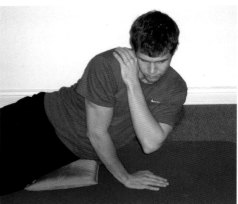

Figure 12-41: Side tricep raises.

SELF-RESISTANCE ARM EXERCISES

Make a fist with one hand and put it in the palm of the other hand as shown in the photograph (Fig. 12-42). Do a curl movement exercising the biceps of your lower arm while resisting with the triceps of your upper arm (Fig. 12-43). Then, push your lower hand down by contracting your triceps of the upper arm against your biceps of your lower arm. This is a good, quick upper arm exercise that can be performed when you don't have access to weights. Make sure you repeat the movement on both sides by switching the upper and lower hands.

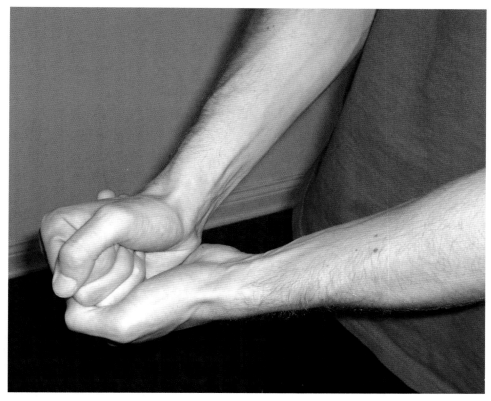

Figure 12-42: Hand placement for self-resistance arm exercises.

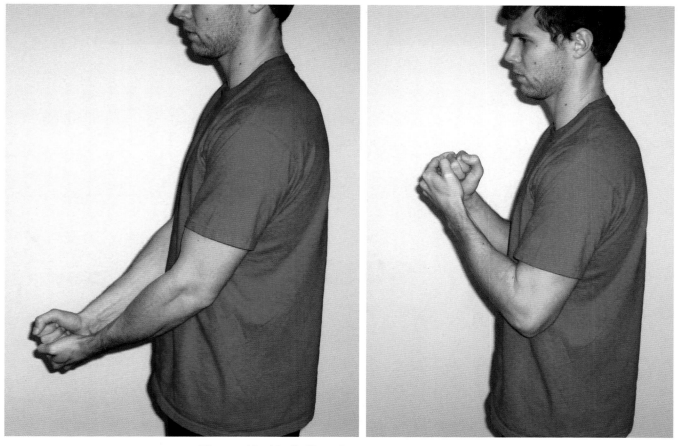

Figure 12-43: Self-resistance arm exercise.

POOL EXERCISES

Swimming pools allow for a quick, effective, and balanced upper body workout. Water resistance increases with the speed of movement, and you can put your fingers together to create even more resistance. The three pool exercises that follow are a quick and easy way to exercise the major muscle groups of the upper body.

FRONT/REVERSE FLIES

Standing with the water at shoulder level, move your arms forward like you are doing dumbbell flies to exercise your chest, and backward like reverse flies to exercise your back (Fig. 12-44). This exercise rapidly works the antagonistic muscles in your chest and upper back.

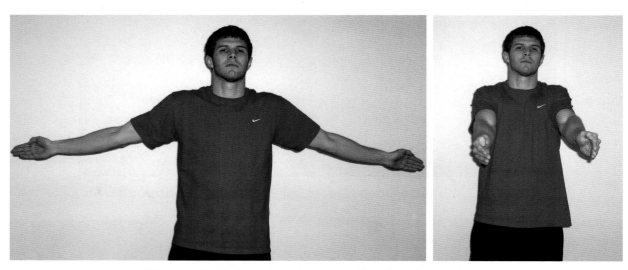

Figure 12-44: Front and reverse flies (pool exercise).

LATERAL RAISES/ARM ADDUCTION

Lift your arms to shoulder level like you are doing lateral dumbbell raises and then push them down to your side (Fig. 12-45). This is a great workout for the shoulder and latissimus muscles.

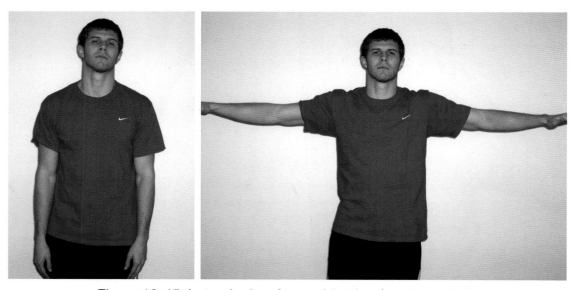

Figure 12-45: Lateral raises/arm adduction (pool exercise).

BICEP/TRICEP CURLS

Move your hands upward in a curling motion and then force them down using your triceps (Fig. 12-46). Doing this exercise with your palms up places more resistance on your arm flexors, while doing it with your palms down emphasizes a tricep workout.

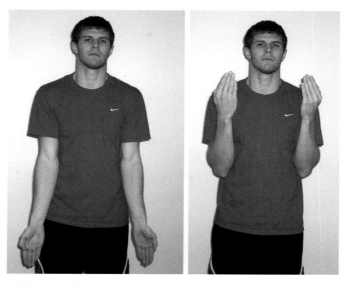

Figure 12-46: Bicep/tricep curls (pool exercise).

STRETCHING EXERCISES

Stretching exercises performed after each exercise session have many benefits, including increased flexibility, improved range of motion, and better posture. Greater flexibility can enhance performance and prevent injuries. It is best to stretch immediately after an exercise session, when your muscles are warm and more receptive to stretching. Hold each stretch for at least thirty seconds. You should stretch until you feel tension, not pain. Make sure you stretch both sides of your body equally. I've included my favorite stretches below.

BAR HANG

Grasp an overhead pull-up bar with a close grip and let gravity stretch the muscles of your shoulders and back (Fig. 12-47).

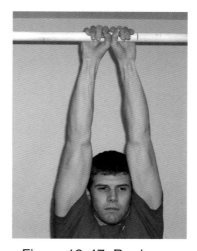

Figure 12-47: Bar hang.

ABDOMINAL STRETCH

Lie prone, with your arms extended under you to stretch your abs (Fig. 12-48).

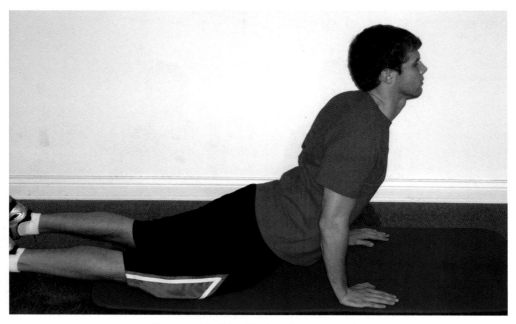

Figure 12-48: Abdominal stretch.

QUADRICEPS STRETCH

Grasp the heel of one foot and lift the heel as far as possible, stretching the quadriceps (Fig. 12-49). It may be helpful to hold on to something with the other hand to maintain your balance.

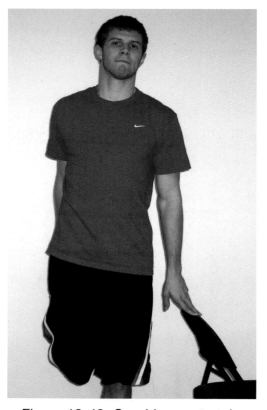

Figure 12-49: Quadriceps stretch.

ONE-LEG HAMSTRING STRETCH

Sit on the floor with one leg extended and the sole of your other leg placed against the extended one (Fig. 12-50). Lean forward to extend the hamstring muscles and hold.

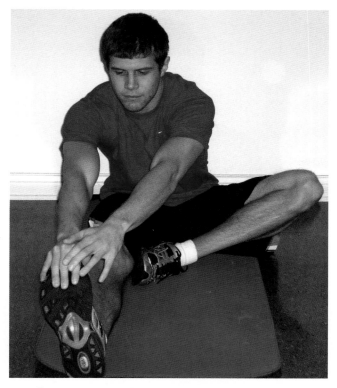

Figure 12-50: One-leg hamstring stretch.

HIP FLEXOR STRETCH

Lying on your back, use your arms to bring one knee toward your chest. At the same time, press your back into the floor (Fig. 12-51).

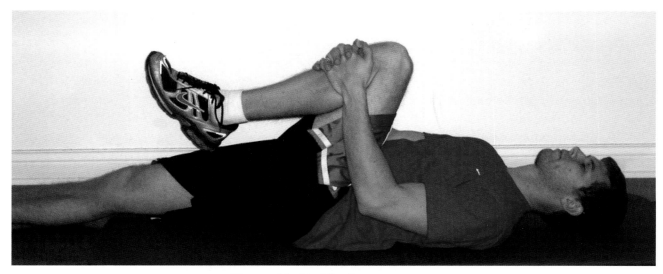

Figure 12-51: Hip flexor stretch.

SITTING GROIN STRETCH

Sit with the soles of your feet touching and the knees pointing outward (Fig. 12-51). For more of a stretch, gently push your legs downward with your elbows.

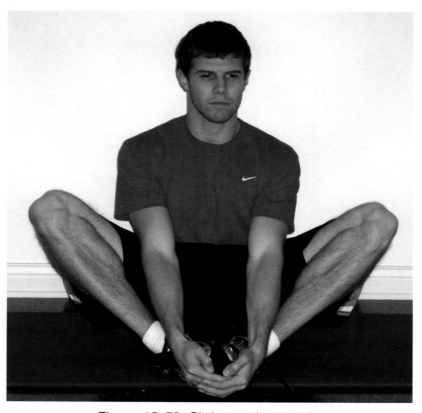

Figure 12-52: Sitting groin stretch.

TWO-LEG HAMSTRING STRETCH

Sit on the floor with your legs flatly extended and try to reach your toes with your nose (Fig. 12-53). You won't be able to touch your toes, but you will feel your hamstrings stretch.

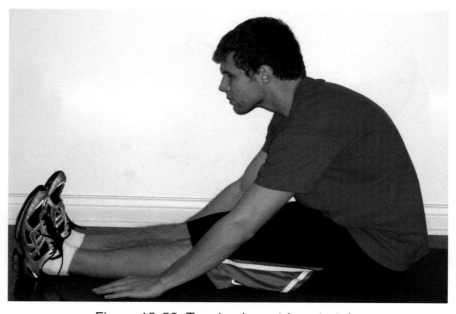

Figure 12-53: Two-leg hamstring stretch.

BACK STRETCHER

Sitting on the floor, raise your legs up over your head and attempt to touch the floor behind your head (Fig. 12-54). If you can touch the floor, hold the position for at least thirty seconds. If you can't touch the floor, let your feet dangle as far as you can go. Don't force this movement, or you could strain your back or neck. Try to relax and allow the weight of your legs to stretch your back slowly. I find that alternating between contracting my lower back muscles to hold up my legs and relaxing them to let my legs dangle often enhances the stretching of my back muscles.

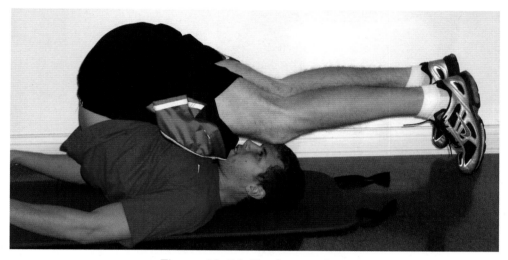

Figure 12-54: Back stretcher.

ADDUCTOR STRETCH

Stand with your feet wide apart. Rotate one foot out ninety degrees and bend the knee, stretching the adductor muscles of the opposite inner thigh (Fig. 12-55). Extending your arms will help you maintain balance—and it looks cool, too!

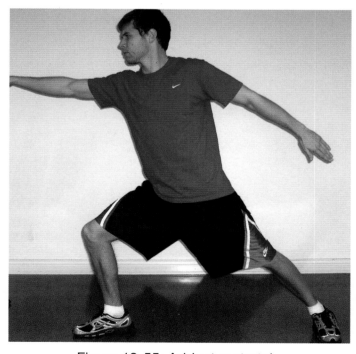

Figure 12-55: Adductor stretch.

FRONT SPLITS

Descend as far as possible into a front split until you feel tension (Fig. 12-56). Hold for thirty seconds. Most people will need to lean on a support for balance.

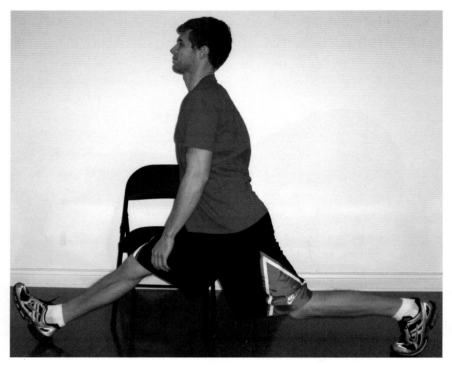

Figure 12-56: Front splits.

CALF STRETCH

Leaning against a support, extend your legs away from the support as far as possible while keeping your heels touching the ground (Fig. 12-57). Hold for at least thirty seconds. In addition to stretching the calf muscles, this exercise is useful in preventing and treating a painful condition of the foot called plantar fasciitis.

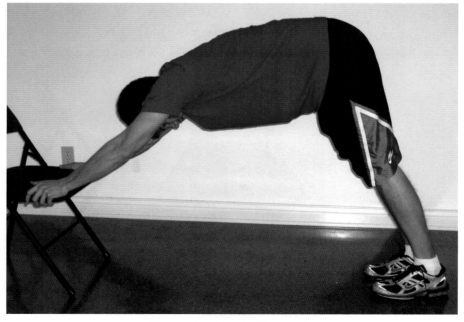

Figure 12-57: Calf stretch.

RECOMMENDATIONS FOR A SUCCESSFUL WORKOUT ROUTINE

1. For any workout routine to be successful, you have to keep doing it. Sticking to a routine is much easier if it is enjoyable and fits well into your schedule. If you are an early riser, exercising before heading to work will not interfere with the rest of your day. Others may find that working out at noon or during the evening works better for them. Do longer workouts on days when you have more time, and schedule shorter workouts or rest days during periods where your calendar is especially hectic.

2. It is important to include both endurance and strength exercises in your routine. Work to equally develop antagonistic muscle groups. Allow time for specific muscle groups and joints to rest between exercise sessions. The amount of rest required will vary with the individual and the intensity of your workouts. While you may be able to walk every day, you may need to rest some muscle groups for several days after an intense weight-lifting session. Start slow and let your body be your guide. If some body parts are sore, do exercises involving other muscle groups. If your joints are sore from running, try swimming or biking. Look at the sample workout schedules at the end of this chapter for some guidelines. A good general rule is to avoid doing the same activity two days in a row.

3. Use facilities that are readily accessible. Plan for activities that can be done in bad weather or when the community gym is closed.

4. Consider travel/changing time in scheduling your workout. A workout performed at home before your usual morning shower may add one hour to your daily schedule. The same workout performed later in the day with travel to a gym across town may eat up two hours of your schedule. Consider using supersets or circuit-training exercise sequences, described next, as part of your strength-training program.

CIRCUIT-TRAINING SEQUENCES

Traditional weight-training routines often have you perform one set and rest one or two minutes before performing another set of the same exercise. In superset or circuit training, you perform one set of the given exercise and immediately start another set, exercising a different body part. Exercising a second muscle group while you are resting the first enables you to perform more exercises in a given amount of time. In general, the term "superset" is used when two different exercises are performed without an intervening rest period. For example, you do a set of ten bicep curls and immediately move to do ten tricep presses without a rest period. In essence, you have combined both exercises into one set. The term "circuit training" is used when the exerciser moves rapidly from six to fifteen different workout stations. The goal here is to group exercises so there is minimal time wasted between sets. Another way to save time is to try to group exercises in supersets so that there is minimal time wasted loading and removing weights from barbells. For example, supersetting dumbbell pectoral flies and wrist curls allows the same weight to be used for both exercises.

Some workout routines combine strength and aerobic training in a single workout session. For example, in the circuit-training routine used by the Navy SEALs, the participant performs five pull-ups, five dips, ten push-ups, and fifteen squats in each cycle. Move rapidly between each exercise and see how many cycles you can complete in twenty minutes.

CREATING YOUR WORKOUT SCHEDULE

Because aerobic training makes your heart strong and helps keep you alive, it is the most critical part of your workout schedule. It should also be the most time-consuming part of your routine. Try to get at least thirty minutes of endurance training at least six days a week. As I mentioned earlier, you don't have to run marathons. Walking is a great activity. Do different activities on different days to avoid boredom and joint problems. For example, advanced trainers often find that alternating between running and swimming is a good way to avoid sore joints. To help save time, aerobic training can be done immediately before or after strength workouts if desired.

Strength-training routines can take from less than one hour a week to many hours per week depending on your goals. Some sample routines that include a small number of exercises each day follow. As a general rule, these exercises are most effective if you use a weight that will allow sets of ten repetitions. As you progress, you may use heavier weights and fewer repetitions to emphasize strength building, or use lighter weights and higher repetitions to concentrate on endurance. If you prefer a two- or three-day schedule, combine days. (For example, do workouts for days one and two on Monday, workouts for days three and five on Wednesday, and workouts for days four, six, and seven on Friday.) If you're also a runner, you may not need to include a leg resistance workout.

WEEKLY STRENGTH WORKOUT SCHEDULE #1: BEGINNER

Day 1–Chest and upper back
Push-up and bent-over lateral raise supersets (1-3 sets)

Day 2–Abs and lower back
Sit-up and good-morning exercise supersets (1-3 sets)

Day 3–Legs
Squat and calf raise supersets (1-3 sets)

Day 4–Shoulders and back
Declined push-up and chair-assisted pull-up supersets (1-3 sets)

Day 5–Abs and lower back
Leg lift and good-morning supersets (1-3 sets)

Day 6–Arm extensors
Tricep press and reverse wrist curl supersets (1-3 sets)

Day 7–Arm flexors
Bicep and wrist curl supersets (1-3 sets)

WEEKLY STRENGTH WORKOUT
SCHEDULE #2: INTERMEDIATE

Day 1–Chest and upper back
Bench press and bent-over lateral raise supersets (3-5 sets)

Day 2–Abs and lower back
Sit-up and good-morning exercise supersets (3-5 sets)

Day 3–Legs
Squat and calf raise supersets (3-5 sets)

Day 4–Shoulders and back
Shoulder press and pull-up supersets (3-5 sets)

Day 5–Abs and lower back
Crunches and good-morning exercise supersets (3-5 sets)

Day 6–Arm extensors
Standing tricep press and reverse wrist curl supersets (3-5 sets)

Day 7–Arm flexors
Bicep and hand gripper supersets (3-5 sets)

WEEKLY STRENGTH WORKOUT
SCHEDULE #3: ADVANCED

Day 1–Chest and upper back
Push-up and shoulder shrug superset (3 sets)
Bench press and row superset (5 sets)
Elevated push-up and spring pull supersets (5 sets)
Dumbbell flies and spring pull supersets (2 sets)

Day 2–Abs and lower back
Ab roller and good-morning exercise supersets (5-10 sets)

Day 3–Legs
Squats and calf raise supersets (7 sets)
Wall squats (3 sets)
Super skaters (3 sets)

Day 4–Shoulders and back
Shoulder press and pull-up supersets (5-10 sets)
Decline push-up and chair-assisted pull-up supersets (3 sets)
Lateral raises and chair-assisted pull-up supersets (3 sets)

Day 5–Abs and lower back
High-rep sit-up superset (over 100 per set) and good-morning supersets (5-10 sets)

Day 6–Arm extensors
Dumbbell tricep press and reverse wrist curl supersets (10-20 sets)

Day 7–Arm flexors
Bicep and wrist curls (10-20 sets)

Try to stretch after each workout. A routine that includes all of the stretching exercises listed in this chapter can be done in ten to fifteen minutes. Stretching is also a good way to cool down before your post-workout shower.

PERSONAL OBSERVATIONS

Only about half of the people who start an exercise program continue the habit for more than six months (4). Long-term success is tied more closely to enjoyment than intensity, so develop a routine you enjoy and modify it occasionally to avoid boredom. My son, Nathan Loy, is a personal trainer who has posted a free series of ten-minute workouts requiring minimal equipment on YouTube called Quick10Workouts. You can also check out these routines on his website, www.quick10workouts.com. Start slow and enjoy your workouts. Listen to your body and give yourself a day off when you need one. Make it fun, and stick with it!

REFERENCES:

1. Myers et al. "Exercise Capacity and Mortality among Men Referred for Exercise Testing." *New England Journal of Medicine* 346 (2002): 793–801.

2. Myers J. "Exercise and Cardiovascular Health." *Circulation* 107 (2003): e2–e5.

3. Byberg et al. "Total Mortality after Changes in Leisure-Time Physical Activity in 50-Year-Old Men: 35-Year Follow-Up of Population-Based Cohort." *British Medical Journal* 338 (2009): b688.

4. Fletcher et al. "Statement on Exercise: Benefits and Recommendations for Physical Activity Programs for All Americans." *Circulation* 94 (1996): 857–62.

5. Leitzmann et al. "Prospective Study of Physical Activity and Risk of Postmenopausal Breast Cancer." *Breast Cancer Research* (October 2008).

6. Coups et al. "Awareness of the Role of Physical Activity in Colon Cancer Prevention." *Patient Education and Counseling* 72 (2008): 246–51.

7. Andel et al. "Physical Exercise at Midlife and Risk of Dementia Three Decades Later: A Population-Based Study of Swedish Twins." *Journals of Gerontology, Series A, Biological Sciences & Medical Sciences* 63 (2008): 62–66.

8. US Department of Health and Human Services. "2008 Physical Guidelines for Americans." Washington, DC: HHS, October 16, 2008.

13: DIET

An estimated 75 percent of US deaths are caused by diseases closely linked to diet (1). Diet has a particularly strong influence on the top two killers, atherosclerosis and cancer.

The major dietary factors contributing to atherosclerosis are summarized in Table 13A.

TABLE 13A
HOW DIETARY FACTORS INCREASE
THE RISK OF ATHEROSCLEROSIS

Saturated fat	↑ LDL cholesterol
Cholesterol	↑ LDL cholesterol
Trans fat	↑ LDL cholesterol
Sodium	↑ Blood pressure
Alcohol	↑ Triglycerides ↑ Blood pressure
Sugars	↑ Triglycerides

Low-density lipoprotein (LDL) cholesterol rises about 2 percent for each 1 percent increase in saturated fat intake (2). Major sources of saturated fat are fatty meats, whole milk products, and baked goods such as cakes, cookies, doughnuts, and pies (2). Dietary cholesterol and trans fats also raise LDL cholesterol. Cholesterol is only found in animal-derived foods such as egg yolks, meat, and dairy products. Trans fat usually comes from partially hydrogenated oils, which are used to make stick margarine, fried foods, and baked goods such as crackers and doughnuts (2). Alcohol and simple sugars tend to raise triglycerides, and more than three alcoholic beverages a day can result in high blood pressure (2). High salt intake will raise blood pressure in 55 percent of whites and 73 percent of African Americans (2). Unfortunately, over 90 percent of US adults exceed the American Heart Association recommendation of consuming less than 500 milligrams of sodium per day (25). It is estimated that 77 percent of the US sodium intake comes from processed foods and restaurant meals (25). As a result, it's important to keep in mind that you can have high sodium intake without ever touching a salt shaker.

Most of us would do well to cut back on the salt. However, don't cut back on sodium intake if you are engaged in prolonged physical activity in the heat. Sweat loss of sodium can be up to six grams per work shift in these conditions (26).

Table 13B lists dietary factors that decrease the risk of atherosclerosis.

TABLE 13B
HOW DIETARY FACTORS DECREASE
THE RISK OF ATHEROSCLEROSIS

Soluble fiber	↓ LDL cholesterol
Plant sterols	↓ LDL cholesterol
Soy protein	↓ LDL cholesterol
Potassium	↓ Blood pressure
Fish	↓ Triglycerides ↓ Inflammation
Low calorie density	↓ Obesity
Alcohol	↑ HDL

Soluble fiber binds to cholesterol (taken from food or bile) in the intestines and prevents its absorption. A daily addition of five to ten grams of soluble fiber to the diet usually results in a 5 percent reduction in LDL cholesterol (2). Good sources of soluble fiber include beans, lentils, fruit, oats, barley, psyllium (found in Metamucil), and wheat dextrin (found in Benefiber).

Besides soluble fiber, plants also contain another group of substances that inhibit cholesterol absorption called phytosterols. There are two main types of phytosterols: sterols and stanols. Phytosterols are found in all plant foods but are most concentrated in plant oils, nuts, seeds, and legumes (3). Phytosterols have been added to some food products, particularly margarines such as Take Control spread (1 gram of free sterols per tablespoon) and Benecol spread (500 milligrams of free stanols per tablespoon) (3). You can also buy phytosterol supplements. Ingesting two grams of phytosterols per day can lower LDL cholesterol by 6 to 15 percent (2). While phytosterols are generally safe, it is not recommended to eat fortified foods containing more than three grams of phytosterols per day. Higher doses have no proven benefit and may cause adverse side effects (3).

A diet including at least twenty-five grams of soy protein may also lower LDL cholesterol, particularly if soy protein replaces food containing animal fat (2). Using soluble fiber, phytosterols, and soy protein together produces the most effective results. A study of patients eating a diet rich in all three substances for one month found a 30 percent reduction in LDL cholesterol (3).

A high-potassium diet can help prevent heart disease by lowering blood pressure. Because fruits and vegetables are excellent sources of potassium, eating lots of fruits and vegetables can lower blood pressure, particularly when salt intake is lowered simultaneously (2). A recent study found that high potassium intake was associated with a 21 percent reduced risk of stroke (27). Eating fish rich in omega-3 fatty acids can lower your risk of atherosclerosis by lowering triglycerides and inflammation (2). Baked or broiled fish are more beneficial than fried, dried, or salted fish (4).

Eating a diet rich in low-calorie, dense foods such as fresh fruits and vegetables is a good way to avoid obesity. Obesity is associated with high blood pressure, elevated triglycerides, increased LDL cholesterol, decreased HDL cholesterol, and type 2 diabetes (2), all of which contribute to atherosclerosis. Some successful diet strategies allow unlimited fresh fruits and vegetables. This is a great way to fill up on healthy, low-calorie foods while also losing weight.

While low to moderate alcohol ingestion can help prevent atherosclerosis by raising HDL cholesterol, its many detrimental effects—described in chapter 8—usually override its benefits.

It is estimated that 35 percent of cancer deaths are related to dietary factors (5). Table 13C shows some of the main dietary factors that increase cancer risk.

TABLE 13C
DIETARY FACTORS THAT INCREASE
CANCER RISK (TYPE)

Alcohol (mouth, throat, esophagus, breast, liver, rectum, bladder)
High fat (breast, colon, prostate)
Saturated fat/red meat (colon, kidney, pancreas, prostate)
Smoked/salted/pickled foods (mouth, throat, esophagus, stomach)

Alcohol ingestion is associated with an increased risk of cancers of the mouth, throat, esophagus, breast, rectum, bladder, and liver (6, 7). As little as one drink per day increases cancer risk (6). Drinking alcohol contributes to tumor development through several mechanisms. Acetaldehyde, a breakdown product of ethanol, may act as a tumor promoter (8). Besides the tumor-promoting effect of alcohol itself, some alcoholic drinks such as beer and whiskey contain other carcinogens such as nitrosamines (9). To make matters even worse, alcohol also inhibits the detoxification of chemical carcinogens such as nitrosamines (8). Nutritional deficiencies associated with alcoholism may also contribute to cancer development (9).

High-fat diets are associated with an increased incidence of cancers of the breast, colon, and prostate (5, 7, 10). Saturated fat and red meat increase the risk of cancers of the colon, kidney, pancreas, and prostate (7). The iron in red meat may be one factor associated with tumor development (11). When meat is cooked at high temperatures—particularly when flame grilled or pan fried—potentially carcinogenic substances known as heterocyclic amines are formed (11). Eating lots of smoked, salted, or nitrite-cured foods such as bacon, ham, hot dogs, or salt-cured fish increases the incidence of cancers of the mouth, throat, esophagus, stomach, and colon (7, 10). For example, the American Institute for Cancer Research found that eating 7 ounces of processed meats such as ham, bacon, hot dogs, and cold cuts a day increases the risk of colon cancer by 72 percent. The reasons behind these connections are controversial, but may involve the formation of carcinogenic nitrosamines during cooking or even in the stomach after ingestion (12).

Fortunately, as shown in Table 13D, a good diet can decrease the incidence of most of the common deadly cancers.

TABLE 13D
DIETARY FACTORS THAT DECREASE
CANCER RISK (TYPE)

Fruits and vegetables (bladder, cervix, colorectal, kidney, mouth, throat, esophagus, liver, lung, ovary, pancreas, lung, prostrate, stomach)

Whole grains (colorectal, breast, mouth, throat, stomach)
Vitamin D (colorectal, prostate, breast, lymphoma)
Calcium (colorectal)

People who eat low amounts of fruits and vegetables have about twice the cancer risk as those with high intake (5). Sadly, in the US, only 14 percent of adults and 9.5 percent of adolescents meet government recommendations to eat at least three servings of vegetables and at least two servings of fruit each day (13). Fruits and vegetables contain fiber, which may protect against colon cancer by diluting carcinogens in the stool and speeding their transit time through the colon (7). Fruits and vegetables are also rich in antioxidants such as vitamins C and E, which help prevent cancer by limiting tissue damage from free radicals (7).

Whole-grain consumption is also associated with decreased cancer risk. Like fruits and vegetables, whole grains are rich in fiber and phytochemicals.

Recent studies have shown that most cells in the body have vitamin D receptors, and that vitamin D deficiency may play a role in many chronic diseases including cancer (18). Studies have also found that vitamin D deficiency is one of the most common nutritional deficiencies on earth, with an estimated 1 billion people taking in an insufficient amount (18). Dark-skinned people, who produce less vitamin D with sun exposure, and people with limited sun exposure in general are particularly likely to have this deficiency. In the United States, most elderly people and minority children, along with a third of the total population, have insufficient vitamin D (18). Low vitamin D levels are associated with a 30 to 50 percent increased risk for carcinomas of the colon, prostate, and breast (18). People living at high latitudes with lower sun exposure also show an increased incidence of lymphoma, pancreatic cancer, and ovarian cancer (18). Vitamin D insufficiency is also associated with a worse prognosis once cancer develops (18).

Five forms of vitamin D have been found in nature, vitamin D1 to D5. Vitamin D2 and D3 are the forms that contribute most to human health, and vitamin D3 is what our bodies produce in response to sunlight. Vitamin D3 also seems to be the most effective in preventing disease.

Treatment of vitamin D deficiency is easy and effective. Postmenopausal women who took vitamin D supplements and added 1,100 international units (IU) of vitamin D3 to their daily diet reduced their cancer risk by 60 to 77 percent (18).

Calcium intake is associated with a reduced risk of colorectal cancer (7). The mechanism of this protective effect is uncertain. It is possible that calcium binds bile acids and fatty acids in the colon and prevents them from causing cell injury (19). Calcium may also play a role in reducing cellular proliferation and increasing cell death of tumor cells (19). In addition, calcium intake is associated with fewer occurrences of colonic adenomas, which are benign tumors that can turn into cancer (19).

Plant foods, particularly fruits and vegetables, contain countless poorly understood substances that help prevent diseases. These protective substances are called phytochemicals. Many phytochemicals seem to be very important in cancer protection, as Table 13E illustrates (7, 14–17). Scientists are just beginning to understand how important phytochemicals are to our health. A serving of broccoli alone may contain over 10,000 different active phytochemicals (7)!

TABLE 13E
PHYTOCHEMICALS INVOLVED IN CANCER PREVENTION (7,14–17)

Name	Possible Action(s)	Source(s)
Avenanthramides	antioxidant, decreases inflammation	oats
Carotenoids	antioxidant	deeply pigmented fruits and vegetables
Curcumin	inhibits enzymes that activate carcinogens	turmeric
Flavanoids	antioxidant, inhibits carcinogens	fruits and vegetables, whole wheat
Indoles	blocks DNA damage from carcinogens	broccoli, cabbage, cauliflower
Isothiocyanates	inhibits and detoxified carcinogens	broccoli, cabbage, cauliflower
Phenolic acids	facilitates carcinogen excretion	fruit, oats, potatoes, soybeans
Phytic acid	prevents free radical formation	whole grains
Phytosterols	promotes death of cancer cells	vegetable oil, whole grains, nuts, legumes
Protease inhibitors	inhibits cancer growth	potatoes, soybeans
Resveratrol	inhibits tumor growth, promotes cancer death	grapes, peanuts
Saponins	prevents cancer growth, stimulates immunity	sprouts, vegetables
Tannins	antioxidant, inhibits carcinogens	lentils, black-eyed peas, grapes, tea
Terpenoids	inhibits tumor growth	many fruits and vegetables

Obviously, an optimal diet would maximize the amount of foods that lower the risk of disease, and minimize the amount of foods that increase the risk. As the preceding tables demonstrate, the typical Western diet (high fat, high meat, high cholesterol, high sodium, high sugar, high alcohol, low fiber, low fruit, and low vegetable) offers the ideal breeding ground for disease. Conversely, a high-fiber, plant-based diet rich in fruits and vegetables is ideal. Additional benefits will follow if nonfat calcium-rich dairy products, soy protein, vitamin D, and fish rich in omega-3 fatty acids are included. If you follow a predominately vegetarian diet, it is important to take a vitamin B12 supplement to avoid vitamin B12 deficiency. Menstruating women may also need an iron supplement.

Vegetarians as a group have less than half the death rates from heart disease as is seen in the general population (20). Because many of the vegetarians in these studies likely had low levels of vitamin B12 and low levels of omega-3-fatty acids, adding a vitamin B12 supplement and fish to a predominately vegetarian diet may cut the death rate from heart disease even more. Some studies have also shown that vegetarians have about half the cancer risk of meat eaters (20). Since many strict vegetarians have low calcium intake (20), the diet outlined in the following recommendations could cut their cancer risk by an even greater percentage.

RECOMMENDATIONS FOR MAKING HEALTHY DIETARY CHOICES

1. **Eat at least ten servings of vegetables or fruits daily.** These are the most nutritious and least calorie-dense foods available. Try to eat a wide variety of these foods. With the exception of coconuts, which are high in saturated fat, and avocados, which are healthy but contain many calories, feel free to eat as many servings of fruits and vegetables as desired. Try to include at least two servings of beans or lentils (Fig. 13-1) and twenty-five grams of a complete protein such as soy powder, tofu, or veggie meats daily. Fresh, frozen, and canned preparations of these items are all acceptable. Juices are okay in moderation, but whole fruits and vegetables are preferred; they will have less sugar, more fiber, and less calories per serving. Avoid heavy sauces and fried or overly processed foods such as French fries and potato chips. While the first few days will take some willpower, many people find that they eventually actually prefer the taste of the foods on the recommended diet (Fig. 13-2). You will also feel lighter and have more energy.

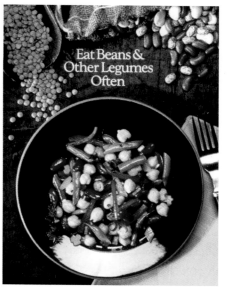

Figure 13-1: Beans are a great source of soluble fiber and protein.
Photo courtesy of Bill Branson, National Cancer Institute.

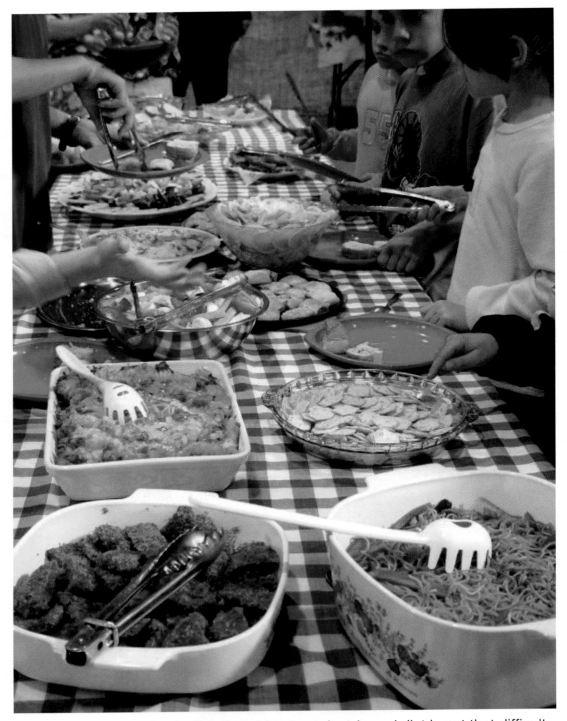

Figure 13-2: Vegetarian buffet. Switching to a plant-based diet is not that difficult.
Photo courtesy of public-domain-image.com.

1. **Eat whole-grain products as desired.** Whole-grain foods such as bread, cereals, brown rice, and quinoa are excellent choices. Choose whole grain over refined flour, as many nutrients are lost during the refining process. For example, in the process of refining whole-wheat flour to white flour, 95 percent of the phytochemicals, 80 percent of the fiber, and 70 percent of the vitamins and minerals are lost (20).

2. **Eat calcium- and protein-rich foods.** Nonfat milk, yogurt, or cottage cheese are good sources of

calcium and protein (Fig. 13-3). If lactose bothers you, try calcium-rich alternatives such as soy milk, almond milk, tofu, almonds, figs, greens, beans, or calcium-fortified orange juice (20). Eat enough of these foods to get the recommended daily allowance for calcium—usually about four or five servings. Egg whites are good sources of protein without the cholesterol found in egg yolks.

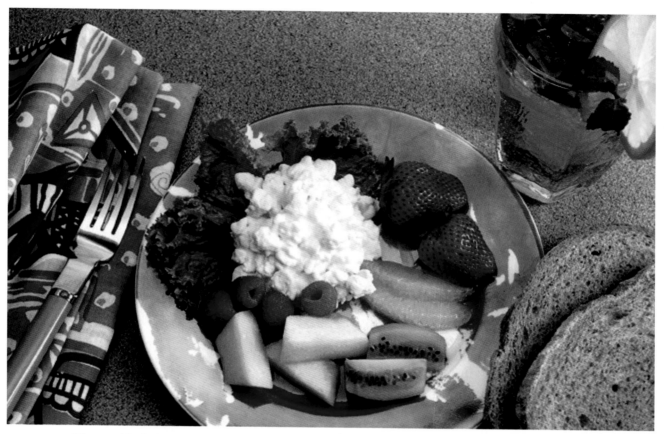

Figure 13-3: Nonfat dairy products are a healthy source of protein and calcium.
Photo courtesy of Bill Branson, National Cancer Institute.

1. **Eat healthy fats.** While saturated and trans fats are bad for you, unsaturated fats and omega-3 fatty acids are healthy in moderation. Good sources of healthy unsaturated fats are nuts, avocados, and vegetable oils such as olive oil and canola oil. The only drawback of these foods is that they are high in calories. Try to eat more grams of fiber than fat each day to keep yourself from overdoing it. Omega-3 fatty acids can be supplied by two servings of fish such as salmon, halibut, or tuna each week (Fig. 13-4). Other sources of omega-3 fatty acids include flaxseeds, walnuts, and canola oil (20).

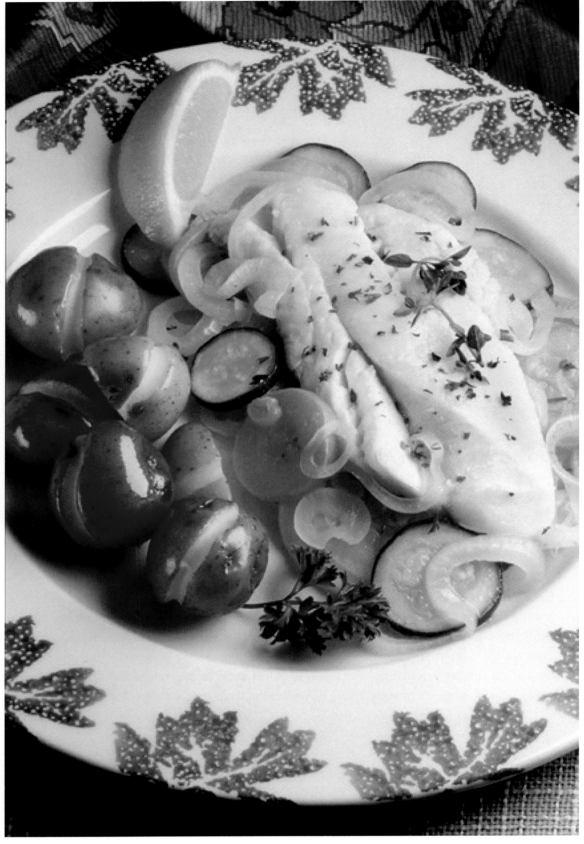

Figure 13-4: Try eating fish instead of red meat.
Photo courtesy of Len Rizzi, National Cancer Institute.

1. **Take selected supplements.** Take at least 1,000 IU of vitamin D3 and 2.4 micrograms (mcg) of vitamin B12 daily. Taking your vitamin D with the largest meal of the day increases absorption and subsequent vitamin D blood levels by about 50 percent (21).

By following these dietary guidelines, you will significantly reduce your risk of the most deadly diseases on earth.

FREQUENTLY ASKED QUESTIONS

Q: What? No meat? That's not normal!
A: True, this diet is not the norm. But we are trying to avoid the terrible diseases that *are* the norm.

Q: I'm an athlete who needs protein. How can I compete with this diet?
A: This diet provides plenty of protein. Many famous athletes, including Hank Aaron, Desmond Howard, and Carl Lewis, are vegetarians (22). Do you think that you need meat to build and maintain muscle? Think again. Bill Pearl, a bodybuilder who has won Mr. Universe four times, has been a vegetarian since 1969. A serious exerciser and meat eater for most of my life, I found I felt more fit *after* switching to this diet (and at age fifty, no less)!

Q: I love to eat meat and junk food. How can I adjust to this diet?
A: Once you become accustomed to this diet, you will find you actually prefer these healthier foods. If you yearn for meat, try some of the soy veggie meat products. I particularly like MorningStar Farms' Veggie Barbecue Ribs, Spicy Black Bean Burgers, Spicy Sausage, and Mushroom Lover's Burgers. Veggie meats are a great substitute for some of the most unhealthy foods in our society. The least healthy restaurant entrée in the US was recently judged to be the baby back ribs at a popular eatery, which contained 3,021 calories, 242 grams of fat, and 90 grams of saturated fat (23). In contrast, a double serving of MorningStar Farms' Hickory BBQ Riblets has 440 calories, 7 grams of fat, and 0 grams of saturated fat. The vegetarian version is also cholesterol free, provides 36 grams of protein, and has 10 grams of fiber!

Q: I don't like fruits and vegetables. How can I cope?
A: Try new varieties and preparations. If you don't like a certain type of apple, try another. If store-bought tomatoes don't entice you, try homegrown, vine-ripened tomatoes from a farmer's market. There are many cookbooks out there that can teach you great ways to prepare an endless variety of fruits and vegetables.

Q: How can I possibly eat more grams of fiber than fat?
A: It's not as hard as you think. Most fresh fruits and vegetables are rich in fiber and essentially fat free. Beans, lentils, berries, and bran products are a good way to add fiber to the diet. Fiber products like Metamucil and Benefiber can be added to shakes, cereals, soups, and desserts. Some popular food brands are adding fiber to cereal, bread, muffins, yogurt, cottage cheese, and shakes. Table 13F recommends a number of high-fiber, low-fat foods, and the recipe below offers instructions for a high-fiber, high-protein, low-fat shake that I drink most mornings. You can enjoy an endless variety by adding different types of fruit and juice. The taste can be further adjusted with low-calorie sweeteners or spices such as vanilla and cinnamon. Made with blackberries, a

full blender provides forty-one grams of fiber, thirty-six grams of protein, and about one gram of fat. You can avoid prep-work time in the morning by placing most of the ingredients in the blender and refrigerating them overnight. In the morning, simply add ice, water, and milk, and blend!

HEALTHY SHAKE RECIPE
Place the following ingredients into a 64-ounce blender:
  1 cup water
  2 scoops soy protein powder (28 grams of protein)
  3 cups of the fruit of your choice
  3 tablespoons psyllium or wheat dextrin
  1 cup of skim milk
  1 cup of ice
Blend until smooth.

TABLE 13F
EXAMPLES OF HIGH-FIBER, LOW-FAT FOODS

Food	Fiber (grams)	Fat (grams)
Black Beans (15 oz can)	24.5	2
Blackberries (1 cup)	8	0
All-Bran Buds (1 cup)	39	3
Raisin Bran (1cup)	8	1
Red Kidney Beans (15 oz can)	28	2
Lentils (1 cup)	16	<1
Thomas Bagel Thins (1 sliced)	5	1
Dates (1 cup)	16	<1
Oroweat Double Fiber Bread (1 slice)	6	1
Fiber One Yogurt (4 oz)	5	0
Old El Paso Fat-Free Refried Beans (15 oz can)	21	0
La Tortilla Factory Smart & Delicious Tortilla (1 large)	12	3

Q: How can I prevent gas with this diet?
A: Most gas in the colon is produced by bacteria, which break down certain sugars, and soluble fiber, which is not absorbed by the small intestine. Drastic dietary changes can give rise to increased gas. Usually the body gradually adapts to changes in the diet through changes in the amount of colonic bacteria. Certain types of soluble fiber, called prebiotic fibers, tend to acidify the colon and reduce the types of bacteria that produce gas. Good sources of prebiotic fibers include bananas, onions, garlic, leeks, asparagus, artichokes, and yams (24). Gradual implementation of the new diet, along with eating smaller portions of new foods, may help during the transition. Products such as Beano, which contains an enzyme that helps break down

potentially gas-forming sugars before they enter the colon; Gas-X, which contains simethicone to break up gas bubbles; and CharcoCaps, which contain charcoal that absorbs colonic gas, may also be helpful.

Q: Can I cheat?
A: Sure, but keep in mind that the more closely you follow the diet, the greater the benefits.

PERSONAL OBSERVATIONS

As a surgical pathologist, I saw hundreds of cases of atherosclerosis and cancer that might have been prevented if the patients had eaten a healthier diet. For most people in the Western world, dietary changes can be one of the most effective ways to improve your health and prevent disease. Please consider adopting the diet outlined in this chapter. If you don't think you can change all at once, start with one meal per day or one day per week. Your efforts to eat a better diet can yield tremendous health benefits!

REFERENCES:

1. National Cancer Institute. "NCI Health Information Tip Sheet for Writers: Diet and Diseases." Rockville, MD: NIH, February 26, 2004.

2. Rolfes SR, Pinna K, Whitney E. *Understanding Normal and Clinical Nutrition*. 7th ed. Belmont, CA: Thomson Wadsworth, 2006: 819–45.

3. Higdon J, Drake VJ, Jones P. "Phytosterols." Linus Pauling Institute at Oregon State University, September 2008. http://lpi.oregonstate.edu/infocenter/phytochemicals/sterols/.

4. Meng L. "Benefits of Eating Fish May Depend on Preparation." American Heart Association, news release, November 17, 2009.

5. Clifford et al. "Diet and Cancer Risk." National Cancer Institute. Rockville, MD: NCI. rex.nci.nih.gov.

6. Allen et al. "Moderate Alcohol Intake and Cancer Incidence in Women." *Journal of the National Cancer Institute* 101 (2009): 296–305.

7. Rolfes SR, Pinna K, Whitney E. *Understanding Normal and Clinical Nutrition*. 7th ed. Belmont, CA: Thomson Wadsworth, 2006: 465–71, 880–83.

8. Kane AB, Kumar V. "Environmental and Nutritional Pathology." In *Robbins and Cotran Pathologic Basis of Disease*, 7th ed., edited by Kumar et al, 424. Philadelphia, PA: Elsevier Saunders, 2005.

9. Liu C, Crawford JM. "The Gastrointestinal Tract." In *Robbins and Cotran Pathologic Basis of Disease*, 7th ed., edited by Kumar et al, 806–07. Philadelphia, PA: Elsevier Saunders, 2005.

10. Dugdale DC. "Diet and Disease." Bethesda, MD: National Institutes of Health, May 3, 2009. www.nim.nih.gov/medlineplus/ency/article/002096.htm.

11. Cross et al. "A Large Prospective Study of Meat Consumption and Colorectal Cancer Risk: An Investigation of Potential Mechanisms Underlying This Association." *Cancer Research* (March 9, 2010): doi: 10.1158/0008-5472.

12. Scanlan RA. "Nitrosamines and Cancer." Linus Pauling Institute at Oregon State University, November 2000. http://lpi.oregonstate.edu/f-w00/nitrosamine.html.

13. Centers for Disease Control and Prevention. "State Indicator Report on Fruits and Vegetables." Atlanta, GA: CDC, 2009.

14. Guo et al. "Dietary Polyphenols, Inflammation, and Cancer." *Nutrition & Cancer* 61 (2009): 807–10.

15. Woyengo et al. "Anticancer Effects of Phytosterols." *European Journal of Clinical Nutrition* 63 (2009): 813–20.

16. Athar et al. "Multiple Molecular Targets of Resveratrol: Anti-Carcinogenic Mechanisms." *Archives of Biochemistry & Biophysics* 486 (2009): 95–102.

17. Thangaiyan et al. "Terpenoids and Breast Cancer Chemoprevention." *Breast Cancer Research and Treatment* 115 (2009): 223–39.

18. Holick MF. "Vitamin D Deficiency." *New England Journal of Medicine* 357 (2007): 266–81.

19. National Cancer Institute. "Calcium and Cancer Prevention: Strengths and Limits of the Evidence." Rockville, MD: NCI. Last reviewed May 4, 2009. http://www.cancer.gov/cancertopics/factsheet/prevention/calcium.

20. Vesanto M, Davis B. *The New Becoming Vegetarian*. Summertown, Tennessee: Healthy Living Publications, 2003: 22–99, 125, 194–95.

21. Mulligan GB, Licata A. "Taking Vitamin D with the Largest Meal Improves Absorption and Results in Higher Serum Levels of 25-hydroxyvitamin D." *Journal of Bone and Mineral Research* 25 (2010): 928–30.

22. Havala S. *Being Vegetarian for Dummies*. Hoboken, NJ: Wiley Publishing, Inc., 2001: 25.

23. Zinczenko D, Goulding M. *Eat This, Not That! Restaurant Survival Guide*. Emmaus, PA: Rodale, Inc., 2010.

24. Jackson Siegelbaum Gastroenterology. "High Fiber Diet." Accessed 2010. http://gicare.com/diets/high-fiber-diet/.

25. Centers for Disease Control and Prevention. "Sodium Intake among Adults—United States, 2005-2006," vol. 59, no. 24 (June 25, 2010). Atlanta, GA: CDC Morbidity and Mortality Report, 746–49.

26. Bates GP, Miller VS. "Sweat Rate and Sodium Loss during Work in the Heat." *Journal of Occupational Medicine and Toxicology* 3, no. 4 (2008): doi: 10.1186/1745-6673 3–4.

27. Strazzullo et al. "Potassium Intake and Stroke Risk: Meta-Analysis of Prospective Studies: 6C.03." *Journal of Hypertension* 28 (June 2010): p e239.

AFTERWORD

Thank you for reading this book. You now have the information that could prevent 90 percent of heart disease, 67 percent of cancer, 90 percent of chronic lung disease, nearly all cases of sexually transmitted disease, as well as most cases of accidental death, diabetes, and cirrhosis. If the lifestyle choices outlined in this book were uniformly adopted, the savings in suffering and health care costs would be tremendous. Please teach your friends and family about the principles you have learned. The best way to eliminate disease is to prevent it from ever happening.

ABOUT THE AUTHOR

Tim Loy grew up in rural Illinois and graduated from Greenville College. He received his MD from Southern Illinois University. After completing a residency in Anatomic Pathology at the University of Missouri, he did a Surgical Pathology fellowship at the University of Minnesota. He joined the pathology faculty of the University of Missouri-Columbia in 1987 and served as their director of anatomic pathology from 2005 to 2011. Since 2011, Dr. Loy has been a professor of pathology at Ross Medical School. He has published numerous pathology articles and has received national awards including recognition in *Best Doctors in America*, *Who's Who in America*, and *Who's Who in Medical Sciences*.

Blessed with an incredible wife and four wonderful children, Dr. Loy enjoys worship services, family outings, exercise, gardening, and snorkeling.